FIRST, U.S. PRESIDENT SIGNED HEALTH-CARE REFORM SINCE 1963

FIRST, U.S. PRESIDENT SIGNED HEALTH-CARE REFORM SINCE 1963

Ahmed Ceegaag

Copyright © 2017 by Ahmed Ceegaag.

Library of Congress Control Number:		2017914228
ISBN:	Hardcover	978-1-5434-5151-1
	Softcover	978-1-5434-5152-8
	eBook	978-1-5434-5153-5

All rights reserved. No part of this book may be reproduced or transmitted in any form or by any means, electronic or mechanical, including photocopying, recording, or by any information storage and retrieval system, without permission in writing from the copyright owner.

Any people depicted in stock imagery provided by Thinkstock are models, and such images are being used for illustrative purposes only. Certain stock imagery © Thinkstock.

Print information available on the last page.

Rev. date: 09/15/2017

To order additional copies of this book, contact:
Xlibris
1-888-795-4274
www.Xlibris.com
Orders@Xlibris.com
763113

In the name of God, The Most Merciful, The Most Graciousfull

- "It is part of the mercy of God that thou dost deal gently with them. Wert thou severe or harsh-hearted, they would have broken away fro about thee: so pass over (their faults), and ask for (God)'s) forgiveness for them; and consult them in affairs (of moment). Then, when thou hast taken a decision, put thy trust in God. For God loves those who put their trust (in Him)", (Holly Quran, Surah 3, Al-Imran, (159). The Meaning of the Holy Qur'an by Abdullah Yusuf Ali new edition with revised Translation;
- "("From the land that is clean and good, by the will of its "Cherisher" springs up produce, (Rich) after its kind: but from the land that is bad springs up nothing but that which is miserly: that do we explain the signs by various (Symbols) to those who are grateful", (Holly Quran, Surah 7, Al-Araf, (58). The Meaning of the Holy Qur'an by Abdullah Yusuf Ali new edition with revised Translation;
- "God doth command you to render back your trusts to those to whom they are due; And when ye judge between people and people, that ye judge with justice: Verily how excellent is the teaching which he giveth you! For Allah is he who heareth and seeth all thing" (58). The Meaning of the Holy Qur'an by Abdullah Yusuf Ali new edition with revised Translation;
- "O ye who believe! Obey Allah, and obey the messenger, and those changed with authority among you. If ye differ in anything among yourselves, refer it to God and His messenger, If ye do believe in God and the last Day: That is best, and most suitable for final determination. (59)" (Al-nisa, Qur'an). The Meaning of the Holy Qur'an by Abdullah Yusuf Ali new edition with revised Translation

- Those who harken to their lord, and establish regular prayer; who (conduct) their affairs by mutual consultation, who spend out of what we bestow on them for sustenance; (38), Surah, Al-Shura Holly Quran). The Meaning of the Holy Qur'an by Abdullah Yusuf Ali new edition with revised Translation

Contents

Introduction ix
1. Obama-Care Reorganization 1
2. Obama Administration Health-Care System 6
3. Health-Care Reform 11
4. Obama Universal Coverage Victory 17
5. The Health-Care Insurance: Implementing the
   E-Connection Roadmap in Arizona 22
6. Health-Care Human Resources 32
7. The Health-Care Nurse Employments 43
8. Health-Care Budget in the American Communities 49
9. Obama Care Helps Homeless Citizens; Parents Need
   More Section 8 and Low-Income Housing 55
10. How are the Current U.S. President Repealing and
    Replacing the Achievements in Health Care Insurance
    Since 2009? 66
    References 77
    Index 80

Introduction

The purpose of this book is to address a popular debate in America right now. Imagine that you political candidate running for office, and you have an upcoming debate, in which you will be defending your position on Obama Care. Your argument broadsheets are due two days from now, one week from now, and two months from now. What are the necessary steps you need to take in order to effectively prepare for the debate?

The first step is to take two or three days to research the topic. After doing so, you will prepare several papers on the topic. Since 1991, Whitecanos and White performed an operating on not a nomadic system, nor do today's political leaders memorize their speeches, the only way to make a significant impact on the minds of the people is to effectively defend your position in the debate.

Your Subject and Manners of Debate

- A literary debate
- An argumentative debate
- A position debate
- A descriptive debate

In order to be effective in a debate, one must be strong-minded through the manners and measurement of the debate. One must read many books, magazines, newspapers, and journals in order to be well informed on the topic of debate. After building a comprehensive knowledge on the subject,

The second step is to write an effective speech. According to author L. Sue Baugh in *How to Write Term Papers and Reports* (1997), the preliminary thesis statement serves merely to guide and focus one's research. In light of the new information one has uncovered, one may change his mind about his original thesis. Instead of writing a descriptive paper about how new conflicts in America have leads to the proposal to keep Obama Care, one may want to write an argumentative paper, such as a literary paper, a position paper, or a descriptive paper either to support or to criticize Obama Care.

A debate is a strong argument defending one's thesis, argument to government or Oppositions Leaders. How should one structure the argument for a debate?

```
┌─────────────────────────────────────────────────────────┐
│         Speaker of Debate or Chairman Came From         │
│            •  Supreme Court of American                 │
└─────────────────────────────────────────────────────────┘
```

American Republican Party	American Independences Party	American Democratic Party
• Judge One, Court of Appeals	• Judge Two, Court of Common Pleas	• Judge Three, Municipal and County Courts

Right, American Republican Party Leaders
U.K.,
African Republican Party (Farmajo) France, Les
  African Democratic Party
France, La Republique en Marche (LREM)
U.K., The Conservatives

Left, American Democratic Party Oppositions
Labour Party
Republicains (LR)

Bottom, American Independences Party Oppositions
U.K. Liberal Democrats Party
France, Front National (FN)
African Youth Party

Preparation

The following are components of public communication and debate:
- *"Assertion.* A claim or statement that needs to be proven or explained. Americans Resolution Home Health Care Attending. Though, Academies is good for America's poorest families like mine to supporting it.
- *Reason.* The act of proving an assertion by explaining, describing, and elaborating between America's Republican Party and America's Democratic Party.
- *Evidences.* Facts, information, or observation present in support of an assertion. Structures show that playing video games causes children to become more violent in personality, because of luck of Health Care.
- Jokes of the Debates. What is a pirate's favorite letter in "issues for debate in Obama Care?" (YouTube, 2017).

This book will debate the issues surrounding Obama Care. The Obama Care was first implemented in 2010, but, new U.S President, Donald Trump is going to repeal and replace with another insurance policy that will help America's poorest people and its middle class people,

In her book, entitled *Issues for Debate in American Public Policy*, Marcia Clemmitt writes, "Today, after almost a century of trying; today, after over a year of debate; today, after all the votes have been tallied—health insurance reform becomes law in the United States of America" (2003, 375). She repeated these words in an address at the Whitecanos and White signing ceremony on March 23, 2010.

Correspondences Concerning Public Communication and Discussion

How much time do you spend each day in conversation about the current happenings of the political world? The average senior citizen, both women and men, spend almost one-hour per day engaged in political discussions or debates. For example, a common discussion may be about the differences between whitecanos and white communities in America.

Abdi Hashi Dhore was my best friend and uncle. I used to sit with him in many coffee shops around Columbus, Ohio, such as Safari Coffee, Caffe Nationale, and Aaran Restaurant & Cafe. He died in 2013 (God bless him in the grave and last judgments be upon all of us). He left many children in this World. He used to warn my children to diligently study the Somalia language. He would also tell me that my children would have a different way of speaking and understanding the Somali language, since they were born in America. They would not experience the same things I experienced during my childhood in Somalia. This would include the way that they communicate and debate issues started in the public Debates in Somalia People. (Dhore 2011 to 2012).

The following is a list of communication principles that my uncle passed on to me. In the book public speaking, written by Stephen Lucas, the author gives an in-depth discourse on these same principles. However, Some of the Somalia youngest lawyer like Ismail Mohamed will be using some public speaking or debate in the American Courtrooms, if God wills to us.

- *"Organizing your thoughts logically.* Suppose you were giving someone direction to get to your speaker. You would not do it this way; instead, you would take your listener systematically, step-by-step, from his/her topics of public speaking. You would organize your message.

- *Tailoring your message to your audience.* You are geology major. Two people ask you how pearls are formed. One is your roommate; the other is your nine-year-old niece. You answer as follows.
- *Telling a story for maximum impact.* Suppose you are telling a friend about a funny incident in last week's football or soccer games. You don't begin with the punch line ("Keisha fell out of the stands right onto the field. Here's how it started"). Instead, you carefully build up your story, adjusting your words and tone of voice to get the best effect.
- *Adapting to listener feedback.* Whenever you talk with someone, you are aware of that person's verbal, facial, and physical reactions. Each day in casual conversation, you do these entire things many times without thinking about your topic in public speaking. You already possess these communication skills", (Lucas, Stephen 2001).

Public Speaking

- *"Public speaking is more highly structured than common speech,* Strict time limitations are always imposed on debates. In most cases, in the courtrooms, listeners are not allowed to interrupt with questions or commentary. The speaker must accomplish his or her purpose in the speech itself. When one is preparing the speech, the speaker must anticipate the question that might arise in the minds of listeners and should answer them. Consequently, public debate depends on much more detailed planning and preparation than ordinary conversation.
- *Public debate requires more formal language than common speech..* Slang, jargon, and bad grammar have little place in public debates. When Carolyn McCarthy addressed the Democratic National Convention, she did not say, "We have damn well got to stop the creeps who use guns to shoot down innocent people." Despite the growing informality of all aspects of

American life, listeners usually react negatively to public debates in which speakers do not elevate or polish their language.. A speech should be "special.
- *Public debates require a different method of delivery than common speech.* When conversing informally, most people talk quietly, interjects stock phrases such as "you know" and "I mean," adopt a causal posture, and use what are called vocalized pauses ("uh," "er," "um"). In effective public debate, however, speakers adjust their voices to be heard clearly throughout the audience. They assume a more erect posture. They avoid distracting mannerisms and verbal habits. Just as the different levels of education, such as bachelor's degree, a master's degree, and a PhD, require more time and study, to improve one's public speaking abilities, one must constantly put forth effort and practice"(Lucas, Stephen 2001).

Attitudes Necessary for Effective Debate:

- Fun,
- Challenging,
- Exciting,
- Daunting, and Discouraging
- Intimidating.

Practices

- Present your speeches.
- Watch your Time.
- Repeat.
- Relax.
- Scout the location.
- Ease into eye contact.
- Recognize your value.

- No penalty for losing.
- Learn from each experience.

However, there was a proverb in Somalia that said, "One finger can't wash the whole face," (Somalia Phrase). In regard to public speaking, this proverb teaches that one must implement many different practices in order to effectively defend one's position.

Issues for Debate in Obama-Care are

- A perception;
- Judgment of the points used such as,
  1. Rejection,
  2. Sustenance,
  3. No point of supporting,
  4. Any questions;
- An impression;
- An opportunity;
- A visualization;
- Organized;
- Strategized;
- Mentally ready; and
- Fun in learning.
- Defend any side of any argument.
- Avoid emotional attachment.
- Do not be afraid of public debate and look over their hair.
- Whenever you lose or succeed, try, try, again and again.

In conclusion, I am using this book as a descriptive Obama Care. I would like to teaching and define the issues of debate surrounding Obama Care right now. Conversely, Obama Care has been functioning alongside and the Democratic Party administration has been fighting since 1963.

However, the moral cost of this book is Bashir Gale. He said asked for me, "Do you permit that allowed to advised to you? And he added to leave those Youth's, because you are not some debate and debate was happening at Tim Horton's, (Gale, 2016). I started to protesters my self. Then, I created a new book, which talks about, what is the debate? There were proverb Somalia Said,

- "Ardadaan Kow kabin Jiray
- Kahiyay Marayaan,
- Haday Hingaada U kata baxday
- Al-Bakhro Ayaan Sii'aadayaaye
- Sumaca ii keenan, (Cali Kaar, 1820).

In this book, I will also discuss the history of the differences between Obama Care, and Americans Republican Party. The different ways that health-care affects or future of the middle class citizens and poorest citizens in America.

Chapter 1

Obama-Care Reorganization

The Obama-Care issue has been debated for many years. Every president in America has tried to resolve it. The issue of health care has long been debated and reformed, but President Barack Obama won this health-care reform in 2009. President Obama's management and contemporaneous federalism created a new law, making the agreement connection between the richest and poorest people in America a public administration in federalism. The health-care demand for payment officially was recognized in Washington, DC.

The majorities of the House of Representatives have been debating health-care issues since 1963 but continue to argue with reference to private health-care companies. Even before taking office as President, Barack Obama had created free health bills.

First, free health care is good for America's poorest people and for the middle class, because many private health-care companies are struggling. Health care had worked in the public administration, but Obama sought equality for all Americans.

James Stacey Taylor, in the *Journal of Law*, makes a case for the purpose of the free market. Stipulation of health care was in cooperation with the free market and well-fare. It should also be regulated with honesty and resonance in America's national government and the state governments. Health care under the free market will create better quality service for all Americans. It will be directed towards the quality and condition of people rather than determined by the political demographics of each state.

These health-care issues, despite Democrats and Republicans agreeing this year to end the argument between public administrations and opposing leaderships, because Republicans agreed not to increase tax returns and the Republican Party accepted the health care, the health care bill will never return to congress. This is a good step towards leading public organizations in the right ways of accountability in the democratic system in America.

Majority of House Republicans had been in opposition when President Barack Obama was elected. These administrations were supportive of the idea that health care could be free in the public administration.

The need of health care among America's poorest people is the foundation of the main beliefs supporting the health care bill—precisely in the judgment in the public administration system, which holds to truth-seeking principles. This also embodies the spirit of the United States of America.

Second, the health care industry has created many jobs. Many people wanted health care; however, municipal administrators worked hard along with big businesses to regulate prescription proportions, According to Kavita Bhatnagar and Kalpana Srivastava, "job satisfaction among health-care professionals acquires significance for the purpose of maximization of human resource potential."

The departments of health care created many jobs and planned to create more in the future as a result of maintaining private organizations as well as insurance companies. Many people could not afford the higher costs of private companies, but health care and health care jobs are still necessary in poor and rural areas. In response, local governments created more health care helped an employment's.

The U.S. Senate and House, which made it institutional in America, had thought the health-care departments expected the federalist system to create more jobs than other departments. Their expectations were met, as many jobs were created over the years. However, on a negative note, bureaucracy powers dangerously looked forward to serving unhealthy people in America. This established more jobs in the American public.

On the other side, the Republican Party did not think of that "discretionary authority." Their management has been the poorest in the public administration system. Before President Obama's term they looked forward to what repealing and replacing his policies in the next administration. They wanted to build blocks in preparation for a potential victory in the 2017 new president in America.

America is a great country, yet it did not have a health-care system until 1963. The guiding principle behind the creation of the health care system was increasing the opportunity for all Americans to have access to affordable health care. Free health care would not have been beneficial to America, because it would actually decrease opportunities for hard working individuals. Affordable health care created more opportunities for people to work and to receive medical treatment.

Even with these benefits, Republicans worked to oppose the benefits of health care. They claimed that benefits would be addictive; they also showed no respect for the principal leaders who had carefully thought out ways to make health care beneficial for the American public. For example, during the war in Iraq and Afghanistan, the Republican Party spent billions of dollars on war efforts but ignored the issue of health care for the common people and still, Americans government no resolution both countries in Iraq and Afghanistan.

During the Obama administration, the Republicans' leadership motionlessly cried against nearly every action Obama took. In 2014 and 2015, they began to prepare to overturn Obama's policies in the coming administration. At the same time, almost half of the states also did not approve of Obama care, even though it was officially recognized in the national government.

In conclusion, my expectation is that health care will not be annulled. Health care act has helped many people since 2010. However, the current Republican Party may be the unhealthiest party in America since 1774. They do not have a plan for health insurance. Yet health insurance companies report that many students, members of the poorest communities, those in the army, and the immigrants still have no insurance. This makes it clear that health insurance is more necessary than what Republican leaders are willing to admit.

Chapter 2

Obama Administration Health-Care System

First, U.S. President Signed Health-Care Reform Since 1963

The first time the Democratic Party proposed a new health care system, in 1963, the Republican Party said Medicade and Medicare were better, and health care. However, in 2010, the majority of the House, which was from the Democratic Party, reformed health care policies for the first time since 1963, but they did not make as great an impact as they had originally thought.

Both sides argued with each other over which way to steer the future of America's interest. In response President Obama threatened, "I will shut down the U.S government." He planned to use the veto against the strategy of the Republican Party, which kept the Republicans from caring out their plans.

For two weeks, the U.S government shut down while the Republican Party leaders had Appealed against the health-cares bills, including government bills. The majority of Republicans were in disagreement with it, insisting that it was a waste of time and money. They wanted to overthrow the Obama Care bills but could not do so during Obama's time in office.

What are the chief designations of the challenging and distinguishing applications of Obama Care? The U.S government faced numerous problems when the Obama administration ordered the two-week shutdown. The shutdown increased the national debt to $16.7 trillion. Had the shutdown gone till October 17, 2013, the debt would have increased tremendously to $17.5 trillion. However, to avoid such calamity, the GOP allowed the president a full vote and the government restarted.

In 2014, the Grand Old Party (GOP) representatives did not allow a trusting public policy and health-care bill to the public, and the Republicans won decriminalized bills. Because numerous GOPs worried about health contracts within health care that would follow, the United States' partnership of representatives started debating over future bills.

At the same time, the Obama administration faced three problems: first, the destruction of Syria's chemical weapons; second, the U.S government was shut down for two weeks; and third, the health-care website experienced technical difficulties, the reason of which the White and Whitecanos House did not provide a convincing answer. The website was designed for 50,000 or 70,000 users that time, but the site crashed when 250,000 people tried to sign up for health-care insurance. The President, speaking on this matter, said, "We will fix the problems as soon as we can".

On the MSNBC television network, Meredith Clark said that House Minority spearhead Nancy Pelosi met with the Republicans, during the shutdown period, to deal with the issue of healthcare and to talk about restarting the government.

On the other hand, NBC's Kristen Welker said she did not know if Americans could pay for insurance or if uninsured Americans could not understand health-care. She concluded that it would take time for both government parties to organize their plans.

Some time ago, Medicare had a customary insurance for the higher-level memberships, but it principally sheltered the high-class people, who could pay for medical care, from the lowest class. At first, doctors and hospitals accepted only patients who had medical insurance, but now, the government has pushed them to also accept welfare patients.

Americans indicated support for the new system of Obama Care, which sequestered health care to be developed and to be regenerated in a decent technique.

What is Obama recommending for health-care resolution? Obama planned for the Medicaid and Medicare patients to automatically receive Obama Care. These companies would then never deliver new health care contracts.

For the historical first years of intellectual the Grand Old Party GOP, they will respect Obama Care in 2017. Why? The health care will be constricts have the GOP, and GOPs feared that point when the Grand Old Party will be giving the Democratic Party support in the future.

The Republicans struggled to believe that Obama Care is better than Medicaid, but they are willing to get private insurance from

Obama Care. For these reasons, the Republicans decided to shut down the government for two weeks.

However, Obama Care is cheaper than Medicare and Medicaid insurance. The biggest challenge for the Republican Party will be ending Obama Care without question. They also suffered big losses in the House of Representatives in 2014.

Author Chris Cillizza of *Washington Post* writes that the Republican Party fails to appeal to the shifting demographics of our country. Many of the young White and Whitecanos are looking for opportunities and jobs and will support the party that offers the most hope for their futures.

In the future, health care will be against Medicare and Medicaid's waiver in businesses, and that is why Republicans are opposed to it, since many people are registered with Medicaid. Furthermore, Obama Care covers prescription drugs and will, which is why many people signed up for it. Obama Care will also include dental treatment, and everyone is eligible for Obama Care.

After the website crashed, the Obama administration perfected their advertisements, communicating to all organizations that could use Obama Care. Free health care will make it easier for young and old people alike to access medical care, similar to the system in the United Kingdom and the European Union. This, in return, will promote health care and improve jobs for all, and the United States will attract more people who will take advantage of this program.

In conclusion, Obama care will establish new health care organizations alongside Medicade and Medicare. These companies owned the market and have been able to protect their own interests since 1963. This is why these companies and the Republican party are against Obama care. They are not interested in change for the future.

Chapter 3

Health-Care Reform

Health care has become more effective over the years. Early in my childhood, medicine became a necessity in America. Medicines were not helping American, poor citizens and the middle class, but it helped richest citizens in America. However, Health care has become part of federal unions and state welfares.

However, the cost of medicine has limited low-income and middle class families, and eligibility requirements into government programs. According to Marcia Clemmitt (2003, 375), who wrote a book called *Issues for Debate in American Public Policy*, "Today, after almost a century of trying; today, after over a year of debate; today, after all the votes have been tallied—health insurance reform becomes law in the United States of America." This was proclaimed at the White House signing ceremony on March 23, 2010.

A long time ago, Medicare had been a standard cover for the upper class, but today, it mainly covers the lower class, which can pay Medicare repayment for doctors and hospitals.

For example, in 2016, American chose new president in the White House, who supported Medicare and private health-care planning. They have not liked health care. According to Marcia Clemmitt (2003, 376). It's means institutions and experiments that policymakers hope can eventually lower health-care costs, says Michael E. Clemmitt, a professor in a medical school.

Each statement has different opinions, and I did not agree with the professor's program to go against the U.S president because the president could do a federal benefit to every person, which is legal. Again, President Barack Obama said in his State of the Union Address about health care on CNN: "Greatness requires not only an educated person but healthy people.... In addition, regional medical centers can provide the most advanced diagnosis and treatment for heart disease and cancer and stroke and other major diseases."

This means that first, over the next decade; socialization will be needed in America's health care and educational system. American families will also need the federal government to keep health care alive. For the period of my first few years of scholarly study, I had a lot of difficulty getting medical insurance because private insurance is more expensive than public insurance. The government must legalize health care for everyone and provide easy access to it.

The biggest problem between Republicans and Democratic was when they suffered big losses in the House of Representatives in 2010. According to CNN, "health care isn't a recent hot-button issue for Americans. Shortly after President Lyndon B. Johnson's fight to introduce his Medicare program, he spoke of it during his State of the Union Address in 1966: 'I frequently feel as if I were studying the disparagement of others, not including really developed American people.'"

Each student has had different problems with eligibility for health care in their first year in school. Because of this, a third person would have to apply for medical insurance for the student. Medical insurance is saving more money for everyone.

Home Health-Care Restructuring

If the Republicans had repealed President Obama's legislative accomplishment, health-care reforms would not have achieved anything! However, President Obama vetoed the opposing plan, and the health-care bill was legalized in the United States. Because several people were worried about training health care workers, the United States House of Representatives started debating about health care.

In 2014, the Democrats was against repealing and replacing the health care arrangement. On the other side, the majority of Republicans wanted to repeal the arrangement, claiming "[t]he landmark law will extend coverage to about 32 million of the nation's 45 million uninsured people by: Expanding Medicaid; Providing subsidies to help low-and middle-income families by insurance; Creating regulated insurance markets where people without employer-sponsored insurance can buy subsidized coverage; and using Medicare's economic clout to cut health care costs" (Clemmitt 2003, 375).

Health care is based on the principles of rights in the ruling, philosophical ideals, and the spirit of America. Health care is going to consequently not support by insurance companies. Especially in America's rural areas, people need affordable and high quality health care insurance.

We are providing subsidies to help near-to-the-ground and middle-income families that cannot purchase insurance because the government obtained care of them. According to the website Brookings, the memo to the President about reforming health care reads: "SCHIP reauthorization—SCHIP expires March 31. Re-authorization is certain; its form is not. Congress is set to pass legislation similar to bills approved last year, which President Bush twice vetoed. Congress may add a few new elements, such as benefits for legal immigrant children and pregnant women and financial incentives to cover children eligible for Medicaid. This bill will pass quickly" (1).

American's young college graduates will generate a low-regulated insurance marketplace for Americans when people do not have any jobs. According to *Issues for Debate in American Public Policy*, "within poison, Republicans unanimously rejected the landmark Patient Protection and Affordable Health Care Act, refusing to ward it even a single vote" (Clemmitt 2003, 375). This means that parties had constantly been in disagreement over the issue of health care.

The Republicans have not regarded the building-block achievement as useful in our public policy. They do not believe it would not be useful to citizens, but rather that insurance could be addictive and damaging, drawing on the heart and brain harmful effects. They wanted Obama care to disappear from America.

America's poor and middle class citizens have a significant influence on the economy; these people will be the topic of conversation happening among political leaders. Health care will create jobs and promote work and a boost in the economy.

The Democratic Party has the strongest government, but they cannot pass their proposed bills without support from the other parties. Most of America's youth need health care, but they do not like weak democracy. All these situations contribute to the aggression and fighting in the lives of Americans. These young Americans must have self-determination and find ways to not depend on health care.

Finally, even though Republicans are attempting to get rid it, Obama care is not something that will be done away with quickly. It has passed President Obama's dissection; health care had extended coverage to about forty-five million Americans without insurance, but now it has provided insurance for all of them.

Chapter 4

Obama Universal Coverage Victory

The large enrollment to Obama Care for universal coverage in the United States reflects Obama's tenure and his presidency at the end on January 20, 2017. Will the Republican Party end health care, too in 2017? The answer depends on whom you ask and who won among the 2016 U.S presidential candidates: Trump. However, it is important to understand that universal coverage for America was something many previous presidents attempted about health care since 1963, but new president failed. This effort of Obama's has worked well.

The researcher, Ross Douthat, supported Obama care to be a true winner with a presentation. The fact that, in New York Times, "seven million has been going to signing a health care", (Douthat, 2014). He has shown the need for this program and how long America waited for it. This confirmed the president's claim that many Americans spend too much on expensive health care and don't have any coverage.

The investigator Ross Douthat argues that it's important that we focus on the importance of health care and the debate and discussion on the differences of opinions, though. The Republican Party is fiercely against Obama Care.

They have obviously agreed on the importance of America getting health coverage and are bothered by the enormously expensive health-care coverage that is hurting many middle-class Americans. The Republicans argue that the coverage will add weight to the already-enormous deficits.

Ross Douthat discussed Obama Care and how much it helps many citizens. It could possibly be a lifetime's achievements for Democrats and equally so for Obama. Obama Care will develop more White and Whitecanos supporters, because many Americans will afford health-care coverage, many health-care providers will have to deal with the government if they try to continue charging the citizens expensive and unfair prices.

The broad-minded victory section concluded a quick fix of the web page and encouraged America to get interested and enrolled before the deadline. Ross Douthat, in *New York Times*, pointed out that the "baseline won't be anything like universal coverage, and it may fall short of universality by a much larger margin than the law's supporters hoped," (Douthat, 2014).

One of the principal performers in Obama Care's coverage is approximately fifteen or twenty out of a hundred of its consumers who are not repaying there leading expenses. They are not essentially hidden.

Whenever the emotionless conclusion ends up, it will be the authentic degree of what way voluminous the Grand Old Party (GOP) communities were really sheltered from side to side in the "affordable care act" arguments from both the Democratic Party and the GOPs that support health care.

The Obama administration has been liberating the number of citizens who prefer a "blueprint," but it states that most of them do not support health care. The opportunity—it did not take truthful documents on how a lot have essentially paid. And purchasers don't have the exposure for the pending consumption that they prepared in that first disbursement.

Stretched, and at the verge of overflowing because it reached its capacity, still, Medicare has been an accustomed insurance for sophisticated discussions, but it has worked and strengthened its roots firmly on the ground due to the fact that it was existing for a long time. This is disbursement benefit the doctors and hospital.

For starters, U.S. citizens suggested maintenance for Obama Care. And they have been working on new coordination for the health care of the elderly. It requisitioned health safeguarding to improve and redevelop Obama Care in a well-mannered performance.

Medicaid and Medicare did not have a surprising opposition, and Congress was closer to the communities and more understanding life in small towns across America. Now, Congress votes more in line with their party rather than on an issue. The Tea party movement was hurting more, and equally, the Democratic party was unable to reach their friends outside of the chamber.

The Grand Old Party (GOPs) was trying hard to make Obama's administration fail. Democrats were doing everything to defeat the republic. Obama's administration is spending a great deal of time marketing the idea, ideology and health care directly to the citizens. Instead they should ask for negotiations with the republic and the Congress to pass, or quickly support, or work to amend any flaws they see in the bill.

Author Kelly Cohen worked in the *Washington Examiner*. "Medicaid wrongly paid out more than $14 billion in the last few years to managed care organizations, often for treatments or services that were not necessary, never performed, or were not eligible for coverage." But we will not know how much more Obama Care will cost than other health insurances in America.

With the legitimate target for Americans to sign up for health care in 1963, tensions were leaning from side to side. However, President Obama's regulation was traditional. Health care became available even with a division still underlying the millions of beforehand-uninsured U.S. citizens. Who has increased more tension between the lawmakers?

In conclusion, many citizens have approved Obama Care. Many Americans strongly support it because they believe it has the capacity to create universal coverage, room for covering many, and they can afford health-care coverage—something they couldn't have afforded before. Many children in the upper class have health coverage, and many adults and elders have coverage, too, but many of the youth in the middle class lack this.

Obama Care is expected to change that. It will reduce the health-care cost, increase the number of Americans who will be able to afford health-care coverage, and retain easy-access health-care centers that Americans so often get used to. The question of the cost is still unanswered, but many Republicans would rather have a more expensive health care plan.

Chapter 5

The Health-Care Insurance: Implementing the E-Connection Roadmap in Arizona

The health care insurances presented intensifying struggles for the health-care administration. They tried very hard to quickly change and adopt the new health-care coverage with very limited time and a shrinking budget because they had a great deal of people who were willing to enroll in it. Marissa Hudson, vice president of public/private partnerships in the Viridian Health Management, pointed out that states are in the position to change for the better and have the capacity and understanding if they caught up with rapidity of the change and need of the states' citizens (Hudson 2012).

In 2005, the governor of Arizona delivered a decision-making instruction to generate a road map for the state to follow statewide electronic health-care measurements and conversations among numerous individuals in the health-care distribution classification.

However, Harvard Business School noted that these speeches are needed to pave ways for partnership between government programs and private ones. If this happens, it will increase the likelihood to improve health care and its cost to benefit the state government and state citizens (Applegate et al. 2007).

The subjects of management and modification in the procedure of altering the previous health-care bill's distribution through a groundbreaking public-private partnership and state health care demand for an overhaul of the health-care system and implementing Health-e Connection throughout the state is easy, yet it poses a great deal of difficulties if not taken seriously and without consultation of many experts.

Contract Considerations

The reason companies throughout the United States of America control expenditures of health-care insurance of their workforces is in relation to why the cost of health care is so expensive. Both state and federal governments invest heavily on health care. If something is done to improve health care and reduce its vastly growing cost, it will save the state's budget; every citizen in that state will benefit greatly.

Arizona's effort is undertaken to improve health-care cost and control fraud in the health-care system.

Massive efforts to educate the citizens of the state of Arizona were taken by the state government; brochures were developed and distributed by the state government to inform the citizens to participate, and many private companies and organizations joined in to help, too. The road map to better, advanced, and conveniently affordable health care throughout the state became a reality and something that was achievable.

"Trouble with Champions: Local Public Sector-Third Sector Partnerships and the Future Prospects for Collaborative Governance in the UK" (Brown and Ford 2010) was an examination commanded toward greater attentiveness in the breakdown of the third-subdivision organizations. Their approach to function in health development is not going well so far.

At this juncture of my examination occupation, I commenced to chiefly and superficially underwrite assignments for peripheral agencies incorporating homegrown consultants: Northern Rock Foundation and the Institute for Local Governance.

Advantages

Medicare and Obama Care has been working in Arizona's health-insurance platforms for citizens who were sixty-five or older convinced newer individuals with infirmities. The communities with culminating juncture renal disease (everlasting food disappointment necessitating dialysis before a removal, occasionally screaming end-stage renal disease, or ESRD) to sign up for this health care plan.

Medicare part A. In broad spectrum, part A conceals hospital maintenance, accomplished nursing capability maintenance, nursing domestic care, home health service industries, and hospice care.

Medicare part B. **in wide range, protects two categories of services:**

(1) Psychosomatically indispensable assistances or purchases compulsory to analyze or extravagate a medicinal circumstance and

(2) Precautionary facilities or health care toward counteracting sicknesses. Correspondingly, shielded are possessions approximating experimental examination, ambulance assistances, long-lasting homoeopathic paraphernalia, mental health management, second estimations that were previously an operation, and restricted casualty-recommendation drugs.

- Approximately 25% of Arizona's populace was painstakingly overweight in 2012.
- Maricopa County, which comprises the government principal of Phoenix, defenses third ready of Arizona's fifteen counties of fashionable health influences.
- Maricopa County's 17% tobacco-use degree was disinterested marginally and was more sophisticated than the countrywide normal of 14%.
- Almost 19% of Arizona's personalities are substantially sedentary, positioning Maricopa County's proportion of grown-up corpulence at 24%.
- In calculation, heart disease was the fundamental reason of 21.2% of the diseases in Arizona's inhabitants in 2010 and was the foremost reason of death for natural Americans in Arizona (Hudson 2012).

Self-disclosing throughout expenditures, company's disclosing the highest calculation in a recovered consequence to meet the qualifications of health-care supervision has been determined as the problem unconventionally. Periodically, the particular determination of self-confessions alters upon the singular distinctions of respective illustration; health care stereotypically postpones the shadowing repayments to contributors who, in wholesome faithfulness, contribute in self-admission.

- Forgiveness and former diminution of significance costs (on behalf of up to five years)
- Long-drawn-out repayment expression
- Agreement of particular punishments and authorization
- Well-timed steadfastness of the overpayment
- Acknowledgment of the usefulness of the contributor's agreement and a decrease in the probability of annoyance of a business truthfulness schedule
- Achievable avoidance of successively trooped health care respectful of budgetary penalization and achievement constructed on the released matters

Disadvantages

On one occasion, an inapplicable payment was not determined that it necessitates self-disclosure; contributors were exhilarated to communicate with the Arizona health development as immediate in the development as achievable to increase the hypothetical repayments of self-admission.

Nonetheless, since the wide-ranging disagreement in description, the aggregate and regularity of overpayments that can appear throughout a wide-ranging continuum of contributor manners were challenging to a contemporaneous and all-inclusive set benchmark from side to side to connoisseurs whether confession was applicable. Contributors must establish whether the settlement necessitates a self-confession previously or whether it could be recovered or controlled through a directorial billing development.

- The careful distribution
- The complicated quantity of health care insurance
- Any configurations before developments that the problems might be determined in the contributor's system
- The history of noncompliance
- The surroundings that control the noncompliance

- The administration's description and whether or not the association had a failed trade of health and upright understanding in place
- Distributions applicable for self-admission might be involved although not regulated toward
    o Extensive routine website errors,
    o Methodical errors,
    o Design of errors
    o Hypothetical destruction of state and federal laws involving the AHCCCS program (Betlach and Botsko 2011)

Cost and Price Analysis

According to Sally J. Reel, PhD, RN, FNP, BC, FAAN, FAANP—director of the Arizona AHEC Program (2011), the Arizona AHEC schedule established funds after state and federal source.

The fiscal years diverge through backing foundation. "The federal economic year was September 1 to August 31," and the state financial year was "July 1 to June 30." The overall centralized quantity of $495,075 was approached (Reel 2011).

After the U.S Department of Health and customer service management of the Department of Health businesses and AHEC granted an award. The centralized reward necessitates the agenda's provincial middle classes toward the release of 75% of the reserves with the residual 25% for money making—for example, encouragement for the state-owned agenda. Protraction of the prototypical AHEC decoration was a commission upon coordinative total funds.

Table 1. FY 2011 Arizona AHEC Program:
Federal and State Funding Allocations

- Federal model AHEC grant ----------------------$495,075
- State funds

- Lottery funds (including FY 2010 forward)-------$11,463,296
- Total state- and federal-allocated operating funds--$11,958,371

Table 2. FY 2011 Arizona AHEC Program Allocations: Allocations to the Five Regional Centers

Funding Source Eastern Greater Valley North Southeast Western
- Arizona AHEC Arizona Arizona AHEC Arizona AHEC U.S Federal
- Model AHEC $74,262 $74,262 $74,363 $74,262 $74,262
- State ---------$430,298 $430,298 $430,298 $430,298 $430,298
- Total---------$504,560 $504,560 $560,560 $460,560 $460,560

Management and Evaluation

PPP profited authority and the then point of the Arizona Health-e Connection behind developing the road map. The direction-finding commission of health started to transition after administration and management to PPP, a charitable donation organization.

In January 2007, the for-profit Health-e Connection Board of Directors met for the first time. Like the steering committee that was generated through Governor Napolitano, the board of directors incorporates the all-encompassing exemplification after health care, public supervision, and purchaser assemblages.

Calculation municipal taxation. Following the road map to enhance e-health, Arizona commenced the health-e construction development to convalesce health-care effectiveness and long-suffering maintenance according to the Arizona Health-e Connection executive summary.

1. Safeguarding health communication presented at the argument of carefulness for all patients
2. Diminishing medical miscalculations and circumventing duplicative medical techniques

3. Humanizing synchronization of maintenance among hospitals, doctors, etc.
4. Expanding health-care investigation
5. Stipulating purchasers with their identifiable health communication to hearten countless contributions in their own health-care pronouncements

Consequently far removed, the Arizona Health-e Connection has begun numerous understated assignments to congregate the goalmouths summarized overhead. Taylor (2017) asked every American citizen how the tax credits are compared.

1. Current law (ACA)
   - Take age into account.
   - Take income into account, with higher credits for people making lower incomes (cutoff: 400% of the federal poverty level).
   - Take the local cost of insurance into account.
   - Grow annually if local insurance premiums rise.

2. Republican plan (AHCA)
   - Take age into account.
   - Offer the same credit regardless of income (phase out for incomes above $75,000/individual or $150,000 / married couple).
   - Do not take local cost of insurance into account.
   - Grow annually with inflation.

In conclusion, the Arizona Health-e Connection Roadmap was an effort undertaken by the government in partnership with many organizations and companies, both public and private. It was efficiently and proficiently administered, and it had a far-reaching impact both in the state budgeting end and in reducing the cost for many citizens, as well as in providing health coverage for many without it. Arizona became the model for other states in the planning to enroll the college-aged adults.

The plan was something that, at the beginning, posed a fearful threat but, eventually, connected the millions of citizens around the state to programs that quickly enrolled them for health care. The government and many participants all had profound respect for the effort. Though it was not without flaws, it has worked and effectively helped millions throughout the state.

Chapter 6

Health-Care Human Resources

Sharmarke H. Gaani created home health care; do human resources have to be working separately under the Department of Health Services? It has been independent with good procedures and admirable managements as a subdivision, performing double of its assigned responsibility inside two detachments of the city of Columbus, Ohio, under the Department of Health Care Services (DHCS) and the Human Resources Division (HRD) and the Office of Collective Bargaining (OCB).

Home health-care human resources jobs are

- Post interview activities compiling notes.
- Pre-interview preparation
- Reviewing paperwork of the home nurses
- Planning questions
- Face-to-face interview of coworkers and nurses
- Interpersonal skills

However, Mr. Kristen Rankin is the policy administrator of the HRD/OCB certificate division assistances to distinguish and contribute with associated distribution and speak well on the future and potential of the branch. Imperative to recover that admirable rating in assisting staff, external and internal, the analysis was made by many—together with their employees and home nurses' responsibilities inside HRD/OCB.

What are the Department of Administrative Services and the Human Resources Division in Columbus, Ohio? Mr. Kristen Rankin, who is the policy administrator, noted that it is a branch of the Ohio Department of Administrative Services and Department of Human Services that originate from day-to-day customer service with incorporation of the administration of livelihood development managers. Mr. Kristen Rankin has been complimenting their enormous responsibilities and how well it has done.

Human Resources Operating

Health Care, Human resources have been employing new establishments, administrators, commissioners, supervisors, and managers and have been the subsequent reimbursement accountabilities. Safeguarding the sanctioned reimbursement policies, agendas, and techniques was succeeding in the entire city of Columbus, Ohio. However, the Department of Administrative Services and Human Resources Division agencies have the biggest responsibility in each agency.

New hire. For firsthand hired workers of the Ohio Department of Administrative Services and Human Resources Division, the department vets the candidates and hires them once they pass the background check and confirm or verify the content of their résumés. They also train them once they join the team or are employed.

However, the Ohio Department of Administrative Services and Human Resources Division constructed a discussion with the responsibility of human resources, and Mr. Kristen Rankin, the policy administrator, oversees the employment. They advertise and display any openings on their website to court the professionals. In terms of salary determination, the following had wage determination: hiring, promotion, adjustment, transfer, and demotion.

Safety and training, These are the acknowledging of instruction, involvement, and implementation of the nominee or after the operative; impression of the situation on the goalmouths and intentions of the unit; and safety, training, and analysis of significant, reasonable advertisements and dealings in the city of Columbus, Ohio.

However, home health care and the Department of Administrative Services are a subdivision of Human Resources Division. Domestic fairness indoors and the responsibility throughout the Ohio Department of Administrative Services and Human Resources Division can make safety and training obtainable in the capital city.

Policy administrator. According to Mr. Kristen Rankin, the policy administrator, the publication mentioned new employment explanations and transformations recommended from side to side of the Human Resources Division; warrant that those who are educated of all revolutions in employment accountabilities so that arrangement of requirements might be valued and improved previously in the development.

Calculation. The calculation of each employee's biweekly wage and recital at a minimum a year, plus the agreement takes salary spreads. This duty commands the consideration of the presentation publication policy and the separable underling of their own company. Advocate improvements in payment, policies, techniques, and exercises, and insufficiencies and complications were acknowledged.

Management. The Department of Administrative Services and the Human Resources Division showed new hire progresses, apparatuses, and supervisors' comprehensive association, payment, a functioning administration, judgment documents, techniques, and sequencers. Mr. Kristen Rankin is the policy administrator of the improvements of the compensation quotient, compensation configurations, and emolument exercises and commends the remuneration quotient.

I am exporting and hiring positions to lately generated and significantly changed arrangements, analyzing advertising documents and engagements, and consistently concluding indispensible adjustment to confirm that the institute was reasonable inside the appropriate labor marketplaces.

Warrants. It has shown new hires and warrants from every department and amenableness with significant wages and hours, laws and policies. The Ohio Department of Administrative Services and Human Resources Division have been gathering as a domestic, internal, and national professional bringing them into the city to learn from them so that the city employees will learn in great deal from the most experienced in the world. They will perform their responsibilities well so that the entire city and state function well.

Payroll. The health-care administration also increased employments retaining effort by increasing salaries for most of the employees. The Ohio Department of Administrative Services and

Human Resources Division showed a new-hire salary-intensification budget topic to health care under the Columbus City Council, which should be following each home health-care agency and assumption and the investment administrator.

Home health care would define and institute presented treasuries for enactment proliferations overtime inside authority. It has been working strenuously in specimen organizations. It's significant to communication that this resolve will construct or compose on the fiscal surroundings of the city.

Equal opportunity. The Department of Health Service and Human Resources Division worked an equal opportunity-detachment assignment to campaign whitecanos and white. It's the contribution on behalf of the state of Ohio's Whitecanos and White communities. This is a good civilization—underprivileged establishments and employment to bring into line those establishments with state-management agreement and purchasing prospects.

Sexual harassment. The city of Columbus, Ohio, has equal employment-opportunity provider standards. It doesn't deny someone simply because of the gender or religion or sexual background or classification. The city, however, doesn't tolerate bad behavior from anybody. According to the U.S. Equal Employment Opportunity Commission, harassment does not consume to be of a voluptuous environment; nevertheless, the container enters distasteful interpretations approaching somebody's sex.

For specimen, it is proscribed toward badgering a female besides constructing violent interpretations almost typically to women, though the law does have outlaw, humble, tongue-in-cheek, easygoing statements or sequestered confrontations that are not identically thoughtful.

However, harassment is proscribed as wrongful action when it is subsequently numerous or unembellished. It constructs an argumentative or belligerent employment background while its consequences are in an oppositional engagement pronouncement.

Twelve-Month Assistance Registration Impression

Throughout the 2016 yearly matriculation, old-fashioned you could do the following:

- After your new hiring, you must register for a transformation or degeneration contribution on behalf of you or your children.
- Type no transformations, then your repayments will have been continued in 2016 until 2020, excluding on behalf of the bendable devoting interpretation of our health care's BDIHC disposition and permitted credit.
- Prefer the diplomacies and treatment considerations of your supervisor beside your domesticity.

Paybacks for 2016 to 2020

- Present-day-started 2016 benefit analysis that will have been in resettlement into 2020
- Our home health-care coworkers' direction, vision, and dental
- Additional employee benefits in our company life
- Complementary for your spouse, your children, and your life
- Accompanying your family and your children's life
- Supplementary for unplanned death and dismemberment
- Short-time disability, accident, and critical illness
- In 2020, benefits that will have been terminated as of December 31, 2016
- Conditional for our health-care employment
- Medicinal repayment
- Our action (before you start, our company must sign it)

2016 Benefits Not Amended until 2020

Medical

- Confident HRA, improved PPO, and first-class PPO will have been permanent and accessible.
- Quarterly expenditures will have been snowballing our company benefits.
- Convinced HRA disposition coinsurance and deductibles will have proliferation.
- Heightening our organization deductibles and limits will have proliferation.
- Prescription of the drug-abridged jots and limits will have been accumulative for trademark and no preferred products for our company benefits and drugs.

Dental

- No revolution in transporter or frequencies.
- FSA.
- No hauler conversion.
- Rejection of newfangled postcards for present-day FSA contributors and up-to-date, activated health care insurance are respectable from side to side until 2020.

Home Health Care Not Transforming Reimbursements or Life Insurances from 2016 to 2020

- Transporter revolution after Ohio and lifetime toward our health care
- No design modifications
- Diminution to volunteer existence frequencies

- Change of percentages upon anniversary of our company's condition and underling symbols hooked on sophistication and age of coworkers or group nurses
- Short-term incapacity and long-standing infirmity
- No modification hauler
- Broadsheet-charge intensification to hourly wage
- Correction of our health-care payment upon disreputable compensation and revolution
- Upsets and life-threatening illnesses
- No transformation in importers or percentages

Changes in Home Health-Care Medicines in 2016 to 2020

- Convinced HRA design
- Setup happening besides the out-of-arrangement co-indemnification proliferation from side to side at 10%
- Intensification of complex deductibles from $2,500 to $7,500 or $2,600 to $7,800
- Escalation of deductibles in linkage after $5,000 to $15,000 or $5,200 to $15,000

Enhanced Plan

- In setup, deductibles will intensify after $1,500 to $4,500 or $1,750, to $4,750.
- Outside setup, deductibles will intensify after $3,000 to $9,000 or $3,500 to $9,500.
- Happening network purchases that are abridged and thoroughgoing will have been accumulative after $5,500 to $13,200 or $6,000 to $13,200.

Prescription Drug out of Pocket

- Thirty-generation quantity product will have been in proliferation from a minimum of $25 and a maximum of $50 to a minimum of $30 and a maximum of $60.
- Thirty-period resource of non-preferred variety will have been accumulative from the slightest $50 and a thoroughgoing $100 to the slightest $60 and a concentrated $120.
- Ninety-day quantity and 2× will have been in quotation in a thirty-day quantity.

2016 Undersized Expression and Incapacity Procedures

- Operational last January 1, 2016, the hourly undersized duration disability plants have been snowballing from $0.525 per $10 of assistance to $0.71 per $10 of advantage.
- The 2016 little stretch of the disability disposition will be professional and ready. For example, monitors and the hourly minimum or maximum.
- Damage and queasiness—paybacks inaugurate on the eighth following generation of incapacity. Our health care will be operational by January 1, 2020, the first day of infirmary assistance. It will be yearned and obtainable.

Visit to Doctor or Dental Price Weekly from 2016 to 2020

Home health-care Insurances	Fixed HRA plan	Improved PPO	Payment PPO plan
New employee	$38.41	$75.34	$35.57
EE_1 dependent	$76.05	$151.49	$261.44
EE and spouse and one child or EE and children	$109.25	$196.60	$323.41
EE and family	$145.06	$244.81	$388.49

Dental	Dental	Dental	Dental
Employee only			$10.05
EE +1 dependent			$20.38
Family			$40.49

In conclusion, home health care has the Department of Administrative Services and Human Resources Division, which have far-reaching influences in the entire state of Ohio. The department is responsible for managing the authority and all those strong pillars that very much so hold the city's foundations.

They have the responsibility of hiring and will have their own policy to retaining the experts yearly or in every six months. Home health care will be working with the governance and branch investigation with you daily and carefully in your company. Also, its influences seep into the budgeting efforts of the city and state. The management branch is willing and often has changed to adapt the pace of the morphing world and the modern trend for the betterment of the city and entire state.

Chapter 7

The Health-Care Nurse Employments

Ali Ibrahim Cumar started home health care; needed to hire experienced home health-care nurses to work with you every day. I have been looking for a home health-care nurse. I found a woman who was used to working as a home health-care nurse (Cumar, 2017). If you get a nurse for home health care and have proof of his/her license in home health care, then that is a good nurse.

It's meaning that very a new hire of health-care nurses must involve nurse licenses of State of Ohio. Whether, they corrected termination at the time of the long-suffering plans in the clinic, like health-care nursing homes. In my first underway approach toward my patients, I asked their complications in co-workers' or home nurses' production, "Did you wake up their access undeveloped before knocking it"?

Author Shailynn Krow (2016) in "Role & Duties of a Home Care Nurse," home-care nurses provide medical and personal care to individuals who are chronically ill, disabled, or suffering from cognitive impairments. They typically work for senior citizens who need assistance with dressing, bathing, and housework. Home-care nurses administer medication, monitor vital signs, and educate patients on health care. They are registered nurses, but some agencies allow licensed practical nurses to work for in-home patients" (Krow 2016).

I beheld the improvement of my home health nurses. Have they done anything to you although happening at a sick bay? We did not contact to your professional doctor about those complications.

Our home health-care nurse was disinterested in developing, plus you're unchanging and sufficient in your home-produced conduct. I developed toward comprehending whatever transpired toward our patient.

Our home health care had been a different element of nurses; which regenerates by traveling to their homes and work. She did not visit our patients on holidays before. She used to examine them the next day. She handed me an expression of their treatments and vitals flat, and subsequently, they consumed the hospital services.

Author Ben Sutherly (2015), "A vigorous public outcry against a phase out of the state's 14,000 or so independent home-care providers has set the stage for another conversation about how to improve oversight of another group of providers: home care agencies and some state legislators are giving serious consideration to licensure."

Our home nurses must be licensed or certified in our state of Ohio. They must understand our jobs and administration of medication. If home health-care nurses are licensed and certified, they can administer medication to patients, including intravenous medications. Home health-care nurses are not able to work and prescribe medications to their patients though they can alter a patient's dosage with a physician's approval (Krow 2016).

Our home health-care nurse had requests to visit eight patients every day at daytime, moreover practically thirty-five or thirty patients respectively weekly. On Mondays, our home health-care nurse can illuminate that presence in home-based health, and it happened selfsame dissimilar from that time. On behalf of the introductions in its place of presence-positioned stylishness in themselves and their own car, our company paid for the gas and mileage.

Krow (2016) added, "Home care nurses observe and assess the health of their clients. They monitor vitals and reactions to medications and look for changes in behavior and condition. Home care nurses report directly to the client's physician and family, especially regarding concerns for new medical conditions or worsening health. Some nurses have specialties that allow them to administer treatments, such as therapeutic rehabilitation."

This home-health principle changed, concerning the patients in the hospitals besides our home health-care nurse. Our patients are in the process toward understanding them. Our company had recovered their own hardwearing services.

Our company, unquestionably, and our patients could be thankful and nearsighted as they grow healthier. Furthermore, that type was not a difference among our patients, and we respect that. We were keen on them during the daytime when they come in or out.

They were tasteless, besides a combination of depressed weeks in the highway toward opinion. It's been excessive in the intelligence toward understanding our citizens; therefore, it was tasteless in the approach to the hospital before approaching back home.

The home health-care nurse worked from 8:00 AM to 5:00 PM, usually. In the sunrise and when our business days will open the door, we have our own plan every day. The home nurse must stay on the front because she will start her request before people could meet that day.

Furthermore, "home care nurses provide assistance with simple tasks such as bathing, grooming, and eating. Some agencies require home care nurses to provide light housekeeping, do laundry and prepare meals for their clients, as well as provide emotional, medical and physical support. Home care nurses are often required to assist patients with toileting, getting in and out of bed and transport them to and from the house" (Krow 2016).

However, the U.S government and the state of Ohio should express at what time they patterned their leaning to the generation of patients on behalf of the day. Besides, subsequently, I called our patients toward understanding at what time they can have an appointment.

For example, Ali Ibrahim Cumar said that sometimes, it's difficult to understand the principle of home health-care management, and although significant toward recognizing employment, everybody resides contrarily.

He added that, our home health-care nurse quickly arrived there in the principal patient's home. They were received affectionately, and their patients' husbands or wives requested supplementary communication.

Doubtingly, if they were single patients before who watched co-workers, then they removed hands from the patient's lifeblood heaviness and patterned their kinship and beloved. Subsequently, they communicated alongside her approaching patient. In that way, they had expended their celebration or holiday.

Sharmarke H. Gaani said that, it's the conforming, emergent, and protracted household of brainpower. Additionally, you might simplify the personalities during your home health-care nurse's visit.

First, U.S. President Signed Health-Care Reform Since 1963

Previously, our home health-care nurse had left her principally long-suffering home, and she was going to conclude a timetable of overhauling a never-ending, happy, highlighted schedule among her patients besides traveling and completing the medication that was picked up for recommendation.

In the way they required our home health-care nurse and had her complete it, they controlled and prohibited her from her car, plus prepared her for an appointment for her succeeding patients.

Our next patients will have something like having their blood sugar and blood checked. They must if our patients' prerequisite is picking up medicines from pharmacies. Sometimes, nurses can change if they receive emergency problems, but they can leave it. Sometimes, our home health-care nurse can work eight hours or more than that. Our home health-care nurse has been required to visit five patients every day.

Sharmarke H. Gaani added that sometimes, when we have sick patients, we send them to emergency rooms and our nurse home visited, and our administration following. The home health-care nurse's would not take care of them, but we comprehended and were disinterested in how nerve-racking the situation was. They were sick psychologically, economically, and emotionally.

Author Rita Prices and Ben Sutherly (2014), "Even as increasing numbers of elderly and disabled people embrace in-home care as an alternative to more-expensive nursing homes and institutions—a shift encouraged by the state—consumers have been given little information to make wise choices about that care, a Dispatch investigation found."

In conclusion, oldest people or our patients will need more help from our home health care, nurses, and administration for lifetime transformations besides cherry-picking every part of the phase. Do I indicate my home health care and nurse-controlled patients toward revenue care for their medication or foodstuff? I ruminate: we interpreted that on behalf of contracted, pending, earlier materials. The nurses are calmer and have completed respectable jobs.

Chapter 8

Health-Care Budget in the American Communities

Obama Care is going to help many of the elderly and disabled citizens who have needed caring since 2010. Farta Ibrahim created a new home health-care community, a non-profit organization in Columbus, Ohio. It's one of the several non-profit organizations that assist the elderly in Columbus, Ohio.

This home health-care community serves elderly Americans and new immigrants and also provides other services to all Obama Care insurances, regardless of how long they were in the United States, if they need their services. It is funded by the state, and it also gets some funds from the federal government.

Key Decision Makers and Executive Committees

- *President.* A man oversees the overall operations.
- *Vice president.* A woman is responsible for overseeing.
- *Secretary.* A man coordinates and advises the president.
- *Treasurer.* A woman is responsible for budgeting and auditing.
- *Public relations and legal affairs.* A man advises the organizations on issues regarding legal affairs. He also acts as a liaison for various other entities.

However, how is it funded, and what are their budgeting plans and distribution? This health-care community association is a non-profit organization. It has the 501(c)(3) number registered in the Internal Revenue Service, or IRS. The government allocates a small amount of money (not fixed in amount)—a sort of fluctuating amount—every year, depending on their application or circumstances. Also, they raise money from the business in the community. They give the businesses that support them their IRS number, and they will note that in their turn-refund form.

Here is a standard of their budget designs or plan for a month this year:

Expense types	Budget of June 1, 2014
Salary and benefits	$5,000.46
Maintenance and supplies	$1,099.90
Fees and services	$99.34
Travel and conference	$856.57
Facility purchase/lease	$559.56
Utilities	$229.89
Equipment purchase	$1,400.59
Equipment rentals, parking, and trash	$7,070.26
Service contracts like computers and Internet	$1,889.67
New technology costs	$560.80
Total of one-month bill	$17,488.53

Their third source of income is a state allocation of a small amount of donation passing through Franklin County and the city of Columbus, wherein, most often; the big organizations get the largest stash. And big corporations in Columbus, Ohio, and other cities likewise contributed. They were small in order for them to continue their services to the elderly.

How did the home health-care community design their budget justification and narrate their expenses from their funds? This home health-care community association receives donations from the federal government, the state of Ohio, the city of Columbus, and private banks. This year is $............, but in this research, it will be confined to only on monthly expenses. How much money did they spend each month?

It is processing the independent fiscal year then programmatic presentation explosions to contributions in the direction of needs calculation, service significance, and resource distribution development.

Much of the home health-care communities' service has composed a salary of budgets. This year is $209,856.98; sometimes 8% of intensifications are programmed every June if the community receives more money.

So, this month, the cost of salaries and benefits is only $5,000.46, and it has extraordinarily accomplished such a payment in the people's subdivisions.

The home health-care community workers are people in the administration, perhaps community administrators specializing in sales and who perform best, including employment benefits, which are contingent on the authority engagement insurance advantage.

The benefits may be based on the 401(k) insurance system, a provision on the influence and significance of the person. Those summations might be unimportant, covering on simple basics before it could counterweigh the absent time relative to the aforementioned deserved salary and benefits.

Our community has good maintenance and supplies and an organization with the maintenance and supplies by the end of spring. This time is between the spring season and the summer season. Most of the time, we did summer classes and community activities too.

Each month but not often, something breaks, and they have to fix it, shrinking their services' funds to pay for that service. This month, the air conditioner broke; they had to fix its air filters and the entire system, which totaled $1,099.90 in expenses.

There were other fees and services that helped us. When we were changing room colors and fixing bathrooms and roofs (one side was leaking during the time of rains), it cost us $99.34.

The community safety and security conferences—organizing one or attending them cost a great deal of money, and its portion drains a great deal of the community-allocated funds. The expenses of this totaled $1,099.90. Teaching or attending cultural competence classes or offering one costs money too; the total cost of each is $274.97.

Facility purchase/lease is construction lease. The space the community use and whatever has been used cost $559.56. And it cost us a lot of utilities money for each month; it totaled $229.89 during one month of summer.

Equipment and material purchase for after-school programs cost a total of $1400.59. Other equipment rentals, parking, and trash cost a total of $$7,070.26.

The Internet and new computers, as well as telephones, cost a total of $1,889.67, plus additional new technology cost $560.80.

In conclusion, the total cost and amount spent by the home health-care community association in one month was $...................... This was when they worked with a great deal of constraint and cut short many services for the community's elderly. They provided necessary services like shopping, home assistance, and watching over them. If something arose, they had to cover with that fixed amount of money allocated for them by the city or state or donated to them by the donors.

However, the home health-care community's services are proficient for our community's elderly. For this, home health-care community's services delivered satisfactory assistances and provided for our home health-care community in each system what they can achieve.

Chapter 9

Obama Care Helps Homeless Citizens; Parents Need More Section 8 and Low-Income Housing

American citizens have faced many problems since 2001. However, the pictures of homeless citizens are growing up, and U.S. administration did not have biggest in the principal helped to Homeless citizens America today. This is happening in America. It started shared concerns in the deceased of the 1970s. It participated a significant responsibility in the stylish materialization of pennilessness—for example, a coast-to-coast production among aboveboard and party political measurements are not good, but homeless people will need help with housing and jobs.

The moral cost of the homelessness of our citizen's has been in the post–Vietnam War in 1973, the Korean War in the 1950s, the Middle East War in 1968, Iraq War 1991, 2003 and Afghanistan War in 2003).

However, Bush families had sent American Military to Somalia two times in 1993 and 2006. The family did not explain to World leaders, and main-points, and what for? Those citizens could grieve the American government. They don't care about Americans homeless, and they were not helped those people. The Homeless have lost their jobs, homes, life insurance and Obama care must helped them.

Medical complications incorporating unembellished life cycles and frightening sustenance antipathies disallowed a woman after functioning. This woman had accomplished the benefits of health care on behalf of the homeless in the hospitals; this happened in Baltimore.

Exclusive of Medicaid, this woman's reservation in the workshop won't be intelligent toward the postulate—for example, countless service industries. This woman was correspondingly apprehensive of the prescription, which was straightaway uninhibited before being appropriately reasonable. It would be originally overpriced. This woman was corresponding with voluminous communities suffering destitution.

Homeless citizens live below bridges, beside river areas and tall buildings in the Americans Cities downtown or near a big buildings, shelters, and churches, but where are the Muslim mosques? They did not help hungry people. Obama Care has helped many homeless people through clinics and housing.

Author NPR, Pam Fessler (2011) wrote, "Athena Haniotis, 38, worries about losing her Medicaid coverage. She has been homeless for almost five-years, staying with her friends, in cars or wherever she can to avoid sleeping outside. Medical problems—including severe hyperglycemia, asthma, life-threatening food allergies and anemia—have prevented her from working. She has not been getting help at the Health Care for the Homeless clinic in Baltimore. Without Medicaid, she fears the clinic won't able to provide as many services. She had also worried that her prescriptions, which are now free or very in expensive, would come unaffordable. She is like many people experiencing homelessness. Their health problems lead to the loss of work, then housing. But being homeless makes their health problems worse. Haniotis says, there's a lot of stress. 'You're in survival mode all the time,' she says, worrying about the next meal, where you'll sleep and whether you're safe."

Homeless Chronology in Americans

- *"1978–1980s.* As homelessness grew into a major social, political, and legal problem, advocates won important legal rights for those lacking permanent housing.
- *1978.* Activist Mitch Snyder from Washington, DC, has led a takeover in the National Visitors Center for the homeless, forcing the city to open more shelter space.
- *1979.* Wall Street lawyer Robert M. Hayes sued New York City and state, demanding a right to shelter for homeless men; initial ruling in the case named for homeless plaintiff Robert Callahan was favorable to the homeless.
- *1981.* Callahan died while sleeping on the street. In a landmark agreement, New York settled the case by agreeing to provide shelter for everyone who was homeless.

- *1982.* Philadelphia law guaranteed the homeless a right to shelter, but the shelter is only provided for two or three weeks. Then, the government must help you. As deep recession brought unemployment, homelessness surged.
- *1983.* After more attention-getting protests organized by Snyder and fellow activists, Washington voters passed the nation's first referendum guaranteeing overnight shelter to homeless people.
- *1987.* President Ronald W. Reagan signed into law the McKinney (later renamed McKinney-Vento) Homeless Assistance Act, which became the major source of federal funds to help the homeless.
- *1990s.* Persistent homeless people led academics and think-tank analysts to crunch data in an effort to understand causes and possible cure and led the Bill Clinton administration to step up to its rhetoric on the issues.
- *1993.* Martha R. Burt of the Urban Institute concluded that a shortage of affordable housing for working Americans clearly was one cause of the long-running homelessness crisis. Homeless forty-three-year-old Yetta M. Adams froze to death outside the headquarters of the US Department of Housing and Urban Development (HUD) in Washington, DC.
- *1994.* Partly in response to Adams's death, the Clinton administration unveiled a plan to reduce homelessness by one-third.
- *1998.* Congress revamped the Section 8 Housing and Low-Income Housing Voucher Program to require that vouchers for rental assistance go to very poor families.
- *2000s.* The idea that the government can eliminate homelessness gained strength, but the economic crisis at the end of the decade threatened to deepen the problem.
- *2002.* The George W. Bush administration vowed to end chronic homelessness in ten years.

- *2003.* The administration handed out $48 million in grants to programs designed to get chronically homeless people off the street.
- *2007.* HUD count showed that the number of chronically homeless dropped since 2006 by about 30,000 to approximately 124,000. Service providers began warning of the potential for massive homelessness among Iraq and Afghanistan veterans.
- *2008.* A recession gripped the nation. Progress on reducing the tanks of the chronically homeless halted; Bush created the National Housing Trust Fund, designed to finance affordable housing.
- *2009.* Family homelessness was up by 9 percent, apparently due to recession, with veterans slightly overrepresented among the homeless. National School Boards Association reported growth in student homeless in more than seven hundred school districts. President Obama signed a law creating new homeless prevention and rapid rehousing programs, funded with $1.5 billion. U.S. Conference of Mayors said about three quarters of a group of cities showed rise in family homelessness and decline or leveling off of homelessness among individuals. Advocacy groups launched a drive to push Congress to appropriate another $1 billion to the program for fiscal year 2010–2011", ((Issues For Debate In American Public Policy, 2011).

However, dispossessed gentlemen characterized through six displaced complainants challenged toward shelter. Inadequate shelter was presented, although supervision programs by intervals subsisted toward contradicting shelter in cutting-edge directives or compression. Dispossessed are communities to treasure provisional accommodation unendingly until late 1979.

Robert Hayes, with a lawyer in the white-shoe Wall Street law firm Sullivan & Cromwell, filed a class action lawsuit against the city and state in 1979 on behalf of homeless men, which was represented by six homeless plaintiffs demanding a right to shelter. Some shelter space was available, but government policy at the time was to deny shelter in order to pressure homeless people to find temporary housing on their own. In 1979, Judge Andrew Tyler of the New York Supreme Court (equivalent to district courts in other states) ruled that the U.S. and New York constitutions required that shelter space be available for every homeless man (*Issues for Debate in American Public Policy*, 2011).

Senior Parents Will Need Low-Income Housing Apartments

The Heritage Apartments helped many people from African Union as well as low-income housing. Basro Kulan lived the Heritage, and she 55 years old came to America in 2005, helped her Hawo Hussien 80 years old. The Heritage apartment Community helped many other people, including Hawo Hussien came to America in 1999. She lived with Dakha Ali almost six years. However, Kulan has ten children and all of them live in America today, and she did not like to live with them. She liked to live with her mother. They lived and took care of these Apartment, called the Heritage Apartment Community in Columbus, Ohio.

> "Since 1974, the section 8 Housing and low-income housing Choice Voucher program has been the major federal provider of housing for low-wage workers. Its rental subsidy means recipients don't have to pay more than 30 percent of their income for housing. Through the voucher, the government pays the difference between that 30 percent and the monthly rent. About 2 million U.S. households currently receive subsidies, which go to poor families who can document their inability to rent decent housing. Most cities also maintain waiting lists, some of them years long, because demand for vouchers outstrips supply.

Overwhelmingly, housing experts say, the biggest share of vouchers go to households headed by single mothers, who make up the greatest share of low-income families threatened by housing instability". (*Issues for Debate in American Public Policy*, 2011)

The manager of the apartments of the Heritage Apartment Community, Shirley Hughes helped housing many senior parents. They helped low-income housing, and she well managed those for income housing. She has been taking care of many seniors, as well as White and Whitecanos. She had also took many Somalia communities who were working or not. The Heritage is the best apartment community in the north side of Columbus, Ohio.

The Heritage is a good community. According to the Heritage, within the last several months, some of the inspections have been the normal inspections where our auditors have chosen random units. The inspection that will be most beneficial to all our residents is the 100 percent unit inspection that the owner of the property conducted.

"We are hopeful that once all of the work is completed in your unit, you will take ownership of your home and keep it in good condition. Your responsibility is to call in a work order whenever there is anything wrong in your home. Our responsibility is to fix it or get it fixed. Let's all live up to our responsibilities and keep the Heritage, your home, in great living condition" (Hughes 2017).

However, Somalia's elder citizens are the majority who lived in these apartments. They have lived their lives well, as well as raised their own children, but the parents lived with home health care (HHC). They did have good lives in the state of Ohio. Every child in America throws his/her parents in home health care, and the state government is supporting those problems. The state's supreme court ruled by that culture, and children believed that culture.

According to a website called Somalia Culture, grown children used to depend on the elderly and their parents. When their youngest and eldest depend on their children when they become old or whenever, they will get their own apartments with their children.

Some of the American political leaders have some of the same culture as Somalia culture. However, according to the website's political facts, Joshua Gillin (2017) reported on this story in PolitiFact. It started like this: Former first grandma Marian Robinson just can't catch a break from fake news. First, Michele Obama's mother was wrongly accused of fake stories of drawing a federal pension to take care of grandchildren Sasha and Malia. Now she's the victim of a new round of false reports that claim she's being charged with a crime for doing so since former president Barack Obama left office.

It means that President Obama grew up in a Muslim community in South Asia and his father came from East African communities, and he knew that the elderly and parents respect his mother-in-law or their parents lives with them. This grandmother did not need to house seniors. The former U.S president opened a new gate in American culture. This is a good story that stokes readers and good children to depend on their parents with their own apartments or homes.

Another example is US vice president Joe Biden's mother, Jean Finnegan. Biden's mother, who died at the age of ninety-two with her family around her. According to Karen Travers (2010), "[his] mother, who was 92, fell seriously ill last week and died at home surrounded by family. She had been in hospice care before her death, a source close to the family said." Biden sat somberly throughout the service with his wife, Jill, and sister Valerie seated beside him at the Immaculate Heart of Mary Catholic Church, which his mother had attended since 1955.

On the other hand, Kulan lived in the state of Kenya African Union. Basro Kulan did not like to live in Kenya, but her mother lived in America, and Kulan's mother used to lived with Hawo Hussien in America, but they lived different Apartments.

Kulan said, "All my children are going to get married, and I did not like to live with them. However, when was come to America? I would like to take care my mothers, plus I don't like my daughter's husbands and son's wives to lived with them, and I would like to live with my mother and take care her."

Our parents will need a home health-care insurance, and low income are very important in our lives. They must die on our hands. Parents do not live good lives when they live on home health care. Our parents' respects are to live with us in good faith in our sociality.

It is good for our parents to see their children, and it would be even better for the parents to see their children every day. What should we do? I did not like to live in home health care (HHC), but I am going to suggest to the American government, the Supreme Court, the court of appeals, and the district court to investigate those parents in home health care.

In conclusion, taking care of parents is very important to me, and every person in America. Our parents will need to live with their children, and the U.S government must have mercy on those children who take care of their own parents, as well as Basro Kulan. The U.S government must give a deduction of the tax returns of children who take care of their parents. Though, our parents can't live without the insurance of Obama Care and housing or apartment.

Somalia proverb, which says, Government can't live without taxes, and our parents can't live without their children'.

If you are sending your parents to home health care, your parents will gain mental conditions, health problems, and skin problems, but if they live in an apartment or low-income housing, they will get the best in the world. Every parent at home health care is going to cry in or out. They used to work, they used to pay social security, and whenever they got old at seventy or over, they must get their own apartments to live and their own children to help them.

. Author, Fessler Republicans have promised to Re-appeal and replace Obama Care but have not said how or when. U.S president Trump has said no one will lose coverage. He added, "Almost 900,000 patients are served by Health Care for the Homeless projects around the country. At the end of 2015, two years after Obama Care went into effect, about half those patients had Medicaid coverage." The U.S president wants to appeal and replace Obama Care. Three parties are supporting Trump's administration. What for?

Chapter 10

How are the Current U.S. President Repealing and Replacing the Achievements in Health Care Insurance Since 2009?

First, U.S. President Signed Health-Care Reform Since 1963

U.S. president Donald Trump is going to request fixing his position after his boisterous first one hundred days inside the White House. Mr. Trump had an air of momentousness and discovered explosions of kindhearted support as he delineated a program to reconstitute America's highways and subways, African Union investments. He made no arguments toward China and the Russian governments. The African Union will need investments such as subways, airports, imports and exports, farms, sports, and colleges, and every state government inside the African Union is willing in those ideas.

U.S president Donald Trump will be designating websites through law breaking and pushing for world peace, worsening infrastructure and weakening administrations that the American states have been rebuilding since 1933.

"Unless the Republican Senators are total quitters, Repeal & Replace is not dead! Demand another vote before voting on any other bill" (Twitter, Donald Trump, 2017).

"The very outdated filibuster rule must go. Budget reconciliation is killing R's in Senate. Mitch M, go to 51 votes NOW and WIN. IT'S TIME! (Twitter, Donald Trump, 2017).

"Republicans is the Senate will never win if they don't go to a 51 vote majority now. They look like fools and are just wasting time. (Twitter, Donald Trump, 2017).

"If a new Healthcare bill is not approved quickly, Bailouts for insurance Companies and bailouts for members of congress will end very soon! (Twitter, Donald Trump, 2017).

Because of the rumors that the Russians helped Donald Trump win the presidential election in 2016, it would be in his best interest to stop contact with them.

U.S president Donald Trump's speech must affect his strategies to serve the populace. The health-care system and tax code must have the longest plan in America's history, but it was undersized on particulars, and they were substantially proud to be American.

"Struggling to steer a bitterly divided nation with his job-approval ratings at historic lows, Trump effectively pleaded with the American people to give him a chance and to imagine what could be achieved during his presidency" until 2020 (Rucker, Costa, and Wagner, 2017).

It means that if the Republican Party replaced and appealed Obama Care, U.S president Donald Trump challenged Obama Care only. Both Trump and the Republican Party did not have a proceeding in the jurisdictive achievement on the health-care reform.

It should not succeed somewhat! As President Trump planned, health care was constructed on the moralities of correctness in the presiding. He has always said that new philosophical ideals only replaced and appealed the non-physicality of America, which the Americans experienced. All those that are homeless and the elderly will need health care.

"The landmark law will extend coverage to about 32 million of the nation's 45 million uninsured people by: Expanding Medicaid; Providing subsidies to help low- and middle-income families with that insurance; Creating regulated insurance markets where people without employer-sponsored insurance can buy subsidized coverage; and using Medicare's economic clout to cut health care costs" (375).

Health care accordingly stayed, as well as the insurance companies in the future, but the Republican Party did not have them replaced. What for? U.S citizens' asset required being one in the assemblage as soon as one rustic area, although health care is specifying an appropriation to benefit neighbors of the pounded and middle-income descendants who can't acquire insurance since the management watched them.

The U.S Republican Party produced a low-slung, synchronized insurance bazaar happening for Americans in which individual interest did not have any good jobs. According to *Issues for Debate in America Public Policy*, though poisonous, the Republican Party simultaneously precluded the spread and smudge of the long-suffering protection of the inexpensive Health Care Act, repudiating the responsibility it uniformed in a separate vote in 2020.

However, the U.S Congress has been talking about realty during floor debates. Influential comprehensiveness of Americans, which designated health care, had ceaselessly been a dissimilarity happening in pint-size health care, but I trusted an observation that there, completely, should not be a surprise assassination of Obama Care.

According to the *Washington Post*, some Republican Party leaders supported Obama Care, including House Speaker Paul Ryan and the leaders of the House committees overseeing health care, and wanted to fund the health insurance with something called an advanced refundable tax credit. This functions sort of like a gift card; people can use it to buy health insurance regardless of their income (Sanger-Katz 2017).

Obama Care is going to be debated in America in 2020 and will be best debated in the 2020 election. The health-care advertisement will be decriminalized in the United States since several citizens were concerned approaching irregular health care.

The U.S Committee on House Administration inaugurated declamation-approaching health care. It was, aforementioned, repealing and replacing. While the constitutionalists cancelled the health-care position, middle-of-the-road anti-royalists are inconsistently challenging that.

The Republican Party is going to necessitate the surveyed structure block of Obama Care. It was not good-natured in our public policy in America or in the achievement end of Obama Care. The policy, when improved, should not be advantageous to populations in America today.

Obama Care insurance will never fail or damage those administrations, but they can be harmful. The health-care insurance should continue to be legal in America. According to the *Washington Post*, another group, led by the conservative Republican Study Committee and the House Freedom Caucus, believes that insurance benefits should be funded through the more common tax deductions, which allow you to subtract an amount from your income before paying taxes. Tax deductions are most valuable for people in the highest tax brackets. They are less like a gift card and more like a coupon (Sanger-Katz 2017).

Health care should cover fortification to impending millions of Americans. The self-control grew a lack of insurance. Beginners are contributors of the militia, not insurance companies. They were accommodating to distribute commentary for respective constituents alongside preexisting sickness.

According to the *Washington Post*, "during the campaign, Mr. Trump's official health plan called for allowing people to use a tax deduction to buy health insurance. This is a strategy embraced by many conservatives, who have said they dislike tax credits because they represent too much federal spending."

It means that they are veracious that suppositions are supervised to be fewer and exorbitant. They requested an individual to U.S citizens who document presumptions on not working overtax reappearances. The compensation prohibited citizens whose overstretch percentage was low before the 2018 election time.

Health care shall not honor in advance the exaggerated currently and then be precipitous to the up-to-the-minute American youth, though medicine has transformed a prerequisite in sophisticated America today. The unambiguous will have been happening whatsoever, and technique in Obama health care will be better in quality, concerning concentrated America's poorest citizens and the middle class.

Obama Care will have been amalgamated from side to side. The U.S Supreme Court and administration are not individually particular to safeties of Obama Care if rejected. However, medical insurances will be required to unsatisfactorily low-income or middle classes; the richest people in America will not be happy. They were an acceptability circumstance concerning administration sequencers.

On March 17, 2017, in an article in the *Wall Street Journal* reported by Michelle Hackman, Kristina Peterson, and Stephanie Armour, Thursday's action showed that the legislation, which now goes to the Rules Committee, has become the subject of a tug-of-war between conservation and more centrist Republicans in both chambers, who say it must be revised to avert steep coverage loses. The U.S president will erase the Obama administration's ideas, such as health care for the poorest, self-driving cars, technology cars, and autonomous cars.

Laborious beforehand, Medicare and Medical will have been a characteristic camouflage on behalf of the sophisticated conversation thenceforth and currently. It will have predominant health care, shelters, and jobs in the substandard conversation, which are released in remuneration to Medical compensation on behalf of administrators and infirmaries, for America's poorest should not select front-runners to an employment hip in the responsiveness of Medical and recover every U.S citizen.

Health care will be helping America's richest people, but America's poorest will be thinking about progress to redevelop sophisticated and well-thought-of techniques. Furthermore, they have appreciated health-care classifications since 2010.

It will not correspond, and publication has different sentimentalities. And I, skilled, cannot parallel or finish the teacher sequencer concerning keenness happening illogically in the United States' front-runner; meanwhile, the chairperson should complete a domestic support to every U.S personnel that will need health care with legitimacy.

President Barack Obama's State of the Union address said on CNN Health, "Greatness requires not only an educated person but healthy people. In addition, America's medical centers." This means the principal democratic system in the world will have been needed in America. The issues of the debate on health care will be covering main ideas and instruction in this republic's succeeding times—not replacing and repealing Obama Care.

As satisfactorily as American descendants will be a requirement, each state's new direction forward possesses successful health care. These package requirements decriminalize only health care on behalf of everybody. America thought of stylish society improvement, which I acknowledge is approaching America in the 2020 election.

Both parties will not look to postulate patronage to antagonize the humiliating get-togethers in 1963 to 2017 among American leaders debating and still. According to CNN, health care isn't a recent hot-button issue for the American Republican Party. I habitually sense, for example, the condition I was reviewing in the belittling of others, not incorporating the indeed-industrialized American leaders and American citizens, but the U.S Congress and personal interest are each a corporation.

U.S citizen has spent different feelings forthcoming the presence and competence continuously on behalf of health care and the American people's sophisticated future. As an individual neighborhood, it will have the willpower in the fly-by-night program of the street in Washington, DC. Then U.S citizens should need health-care communication unendingly on behalf of medical care and professional fortification in inhabitants. They should indenture legalized consultants.

I consider that medical care insurance will not be exchangeable as added change for everybody's health insurances. On March 17, 2017, in an article in the *Wall Street Journal* reported by Michelle Hackman, Kristina Peterson, and Stephanie Armour, Rep. Leonard Lance (R-NJ) said, "I certainly do not want to move in the direction of eliminating the Medicaid expansion to an earlier date."

It means that they had functioned for conscientiousness in tight-lipped manufacturers and him in contradiction of health-care classification. This was a selfsame special classification than the one the legislature anticipates. Health care should be significantly affordable care. Disadvantage everything in the permissions, and, yet, the purchaser perception that happens among health-reserve descriptions and their families is riches in American communities.

Buyers will get extraordinary excellence and should be of overdramatically better quality when finished. However, the complaint will acknowledge the expression of supplementary insurers concerned. Moreover, it could underwrite the recommendation of the procurer's single-minded negotiations. It should resemble the rejoinder near public issues and the happening conflict of wide-reaching health care in sophisticated America.

For example, U.S president Trump would like to be acting like the most honest U.S president since 1774. Approaching his knowledge, this man would be elected by the people for the people inside America.

However, America's poorest will need Obama Care manufacturers; besides, he would not maintain the municipality, and each resident would contract permitted health care. Principal management would be happening in sequestered companies. There is a proverb in Somalia that says, "One finger can't wash the whole face."

It means that the Democratic Party would be the toughest management although they could not perform everything. The furthermost undeveloped looked for health care, then they would not correspond to the weak Democratic Party. Whenever they got in the White House, this party would become the weak party. Altogether, these conditions contributed toward the violence and struggle happening in the breaths of Americans.

Author Jessica Taylor (2017) at NPR in her article, "Health Care Plan Championed By Trump Hurts Counties That Voted For Him," "the Affordable Care Act replacement plan championed by President Trump would hurt low-income people in rural areas that voted heavily for the Republican last fall, according to an NPR analysis on data on proposed subsidy changes from the Kaiser Family Foundation."

Undeveloped American health care should not perform self-government, which one could contract, with an open hand, forward in this debate. It had comprehensive health care comparable to the European Union countries. Stylish America would require health care. Responsibility characteristic to an institute would experience health-care direction.

U.S president Trump is going to be a flip-flop against all the plans in the future, as did former U.S president Obama. According to *Washington Post*'s Coral Davenport (2017), "President Trump is poised in the coming days to announce his plans to dismantle the centerpiece of President Barack Obama's climate change legacy while also gutting several smaller but significant policies aimed at curbing global warming."

Furthermore, the performance of Obama Care will not get replaced or repealed. Obama Care could construct to the U.S president, who will get more problems right now. This is not good for the underdeveloped stretch our classes have ended at. The Democratic Party in the House will have good reconstruction on the whereabouts, although subsequently twenty-four times for sympathy, which had disintegrated the health-care bill passed.

"If the new GOP replacement plan does pass—which is still very much in up in the air—the bill would still face substantial hurdles in the Senate. Maine Republican Sen. Susan Collins articulated her opposition to the bill in its current form Sunday on NBC's Meet the Press, citing how it 'disproportionately affects older rural Americans'" (Taylor 2017).

On the other hand, it is reported in the same article that "in an effort to woo reluctant members, one of the amendments announced on Monday evening by House leaders would give the Senate the opportunity to give more tax credits to people aged 50 to 64. However, there's no requirement to make that happen once it passes over to the Senate" (Taylor 2017).

U.S president Trump will not make American people happy because unresolved health care should be instigated and hooked on or removed in forthcoming years. It had transported previous US president Obama's investigation to the poor and middle-class people and what they will need in the 2017 election time.

U.S president Trump chased to bar seven countries in the immigration exclusives direction, and that was against the American Constitution and common law, but American judges banned that order. Trump's order barred citizens from America.

According to CNN's Kyle Blaine and Julia Horowitz (2017), "The seven Muslim-majority countries targeted in President Trump's executive order on immigration were initially identified as 'countries of concern' under the Obama administration. White House Press

Secretary Sean Spicer on Sunday pointed to the Obama administration's actions as the basis for their selection of the seven countries. Trump's order bars citizens from Iraq, Syria, Iran, Libya, Somalia, Sudan and Yemen from entering the U.S. for the next 90 days."

In an article in the *New York Times* written by Glenn Thrush and Maggie Haberman (2017), "President Trump began Monday as he has started so many other presidential mornings—by unleashing a blistering Twitter attack on critics who suggested his 2016 campaign colluded with the Russians."

The chief of the FBI, James B. Comey, did not talk about reality. According to Glenn Thrush and Maggie Haberman (2017) in the *New York Times*, "By the afternoon the director of the F.B.I., James B. Comey, had systematically demolished his arguments in a remarkable public takedown of a sitting president. Even a close ally of Mr. Trump, Representatives Devin Nunes, Republican of California and the House Intelligence Committee chairman, conceded that 'a gray cloud' of suspicion now hung over the White House by the end of the day's hearings."

In conclusion, what was happening to the financial plan of the Obama Care that is derelict on private concern? It will be the up-to-the-minute transformation among political parties, for America had been generating voluminous establishments to health care in the countryside from the time of the 1963 John Kennedy direction of health care.

American citizens are going to get Obama Care to the issues of the poor and the middle class, and it would construct employments and sponsor drudgery toward one addition. Though health care had been functioning with the Democratic Party's administration since 1963, it didn't originate to be the hardwearing, authorized health-care structure in the poorest and middle-class citizens. The Republican Party could not compete forever against many things well, if they did not have partners in health care. However, U.S. President Trump Advises has been direction-finding ruthless way actors U.S. government System.

References

Applegate, L. M., A. Vinze, T. Raghu, and M. Ipe. 2007. "Transforming Arizona's Health Care System: Developing and Implementing the Health-e Connection Roadmap." *Harvard Business Review*. Accessed December 3, 2007. http://hbr.org/product/Transforming-Arizona-s-He/an/808072-PDF-ENG.

Arizona Health-e Connection Executive Summary. (n.d.). http://www.nascio.org/awards/nominations/2007/2007AZ2-Health-e%20Connection%20Recognition%20Award%20Application%202007.pdf. Accessed December 19, 2013. http://www.nascio.org/awards/nominations/2007/2007AZ2-Health-e%20Connection%20Recognition%20Awa.

Baugh, L. Sue. 1997. *How to Write Term Papers and Reports*.

Baker, S. 2014. "15–20 Percent Aren't Paying Obama Care Premiums, Insurer Says." *National Journal*. Accessed April 2, 2014. http://www.nationaljournal.com/health-care/15-20-percent-aren-t-paying-obamacare-premiums-insurer-says-20140402.

Betlach, T. J. 2011. "State of Arizona. Arizona Health Care Cost Containment System. Office of the Inspector General."

Accessed September 23, 2011. http://www.azahcccs.gov/OIG/SelfDisclosure.pdf.

Bhavnagar, Kavita, and Kalpana Srivastava. 2013. "Job Satisfaction in Health-Care Organizations." *Industrial Psychiatry Journal* 21 (1): 75–78.

Blaine, Kyle, and Julia Horowitz. 2017. "How the Trump Administration Chose the 7 Countries in the Immigration Executive Order." https://www.google.com/amp/s/amp/.com/cnn/2017/01/29/politics/how-the-trump-administration-chose-the-7-countries/index.html.

Cillizza, C. (n.d.). "The Republican Battle between Mathematicians and Priests." *Washington Post*. Accessed October 22, 2014. http://www.washingtonpost.com/blogs/the-fix/wp/2013/10/22/the-republican-battle-between-mathematicians-and-priests/.

City of Columbus. 2014. Accessed October 24, 2014. http://www.columbus.gov/search.aspx?q=PUBLIC%20policy.

Chapman, T., J. Brown, and C. Ford. 2010. "Trouble with Champions: Local Public Sector—Third Sector Partnerships and the Future Prospects for Collaborative Governance in the UK." *Policy Studies* 31 (6): 613–630. http://search.ebscohost.com.lib.kaplan.edu/login.aspx?direct=true&db=bth&AN=55309031&site=eds-live.

Cohen, Kelly. 2014. "Here's Where $14 Billion of Taxpayer Money for Medicaid Went." *Washington Examiner*. Accessed June 21, 2014. http://washingtonexaminer.com/heres-where-14-billion-of-taxpayer-money-for-medicaid-went/article/2550025.

Department of Administrative Services. 2013. Accessed October 24, 2014. http://das.ohio.gov/Divisions/EqualOpportu.

Douthat, R. 2014. "Health Care without End." *New York Times*. Accessed April 5, 2014. http://www.nytimes.com/2014/04/06/opinion/sunday/douthat-health-care-without-end.html.

Index

A

Aaran Restaurant & Cafe, xiii
aboveboard, 56
accepted, 2, 8
access, 4, 9, 13, 20, 38, 44, 77–78
accomplish, xiv, 13, 24, 52, 56
accountability, 2
acquires, 3
act, xii, 4, 14, 19, 58, 68, 73
action, 4, 36–37, 59, 70, 75
actually, 4
addictive, 4, 14
administration, xvi, 2, 19
admit, 4
afford, 3, 18, 20
affordable, 4, 14, 19, 24, 58–59, 72–73
Afghanistan, 4, 56, 59
African Union, 60, 62, 67
Ali, Dakha, 60
Armour, Stephanie, 70, 72

B

bachelor's, xv
background, 34, 36
backing, 27
bad, xiv, 36
badgering, 36
based, 14, 45, 52
Bashir Gale, xvii
bathing, 44, 46
bay, 44
become, xii, 12, 62, 70, 73
begin, xiv
beginning, 30
begun, 29
behalf, 26, 36–37, 45–47, 56, 59, 71–72
behavior, 36, 45
beheld, 44
behind, 3, 28
beliefs, 3
believe, v, 8, 14, 20
beloved, 46
benchmark, 26
beneficial, 4, 61
benefit, 12, 19, 23, 37, 68
Betlach, 27
better, 2
betterment, 41
between, xii–xiii, xvii, 2, 13, 20, 23, 52, 60, 78
Bhatnagar, 3
Bhatnagar, Kavita, 3
Biden, Joe, 62
big, 3, 9, 13, 51, 56
biggest, 9, 13, 34, 56, 61
bills, 2, 7, 14, 20, 67, 74
biweekly, 35
Blaine, Kyle, 74
bless, xiii
blocks, 3
blood, 47
blueprint, 19
book, 12

boost, 14
born, xiii
both, xiii, 4, 7–8, 19, 23, 29, 68, 71–72
bothered, 18
Botsko, 27
brain, 14
brainpower, 46
branch, 33, 41
broadsheet-charge, 39
brochures, 24
Brown, 24, 78
budget, 23, 36, 49, 51, 67
build, xiv, 3
bureaucracy, 3
Burt, Martha R., 58
Bush, George W., 14, 56, 58–59
businesses, 3, 9, 27, 50

C

Caffe Nationale, xiii
Callahan, Robert, 57
called vocalized pauses, xv
came, 60, 62
cancer, 12
candidate, x
care, x, xvii, 2–4, 7–9, 12–15, 18–20, 23–26, 28–30, 33, 35–40, 44–47, 50–53, 56, 60–63, 67–75
cases, xiv
casual conversation, xiv
causes, xii, 58
ceremony, xii, 12
Chairman, xi, 75
challenging, 7, 26, 69
change, x, 9, 20, 23, 39, 47, 72–73
changed, v, 35, 41, 45
children, xii–xiii, 14, 20, 37, 40, 60–63
Cillizza, Chris, 9
citizen, xiii, xvii, 12, 14, 18–20, 23–24, 29–30, 44, 46, 50, 56, 61, 68–72, 74–75
claim, xii, 18, 62
Clark, 8
class, xii, xvii, 2, 8, 12, 14, 18, 20, 38, 59, 70, 74–75

clean, v
clearly, xv, 58
Clemmitt, Marcia, xii, 12–14
  Issues for Debate in American Public Policy, 12, 14
clout, 13, 68
CNN, 12–13, 71–72, 74
coffee shops, xiii
Cohen, Kelly, 20
Columbus, Ohio, xiii, 33–34, 36, 50–51, 60–61
Comey, James B., 75
command, v
common, xiii–xv, 4, 69, 74
common discussion, xiii
communication, xii–xiv, 28–29, 36, 46, 72
communities, xiii, 4, 19, 24, 36, 49–53, 56, 59, 61–62, 72
companies, 2–4, 8–9, 14, 23–25, 29, 35, 37, 41, 45, 67–68, 70, 73
components, xii
comprehensive, x, 35, 73
concerning, xiii, 45, 70–71
concluded, 8, 18, 58
conclusion, xvi, 4, 9, 19–20, 29, 41, 47, 53, 63, 75
condition, 2, 39, 45, 61, 72
conduct, vi, 44
consequently, 14
conservatives, xi, 70
constantly, xv, 14
consult, v–vi, 23–24, 72
consultation, vi, 23
contemporaneous, 2, 26
continue, 2, 18, 51, 69
contracts, 7–8, 51
conversation, xiii–xiv, 14, 23, 45, 71
conversing, xv
convincing, 8
cooperation, 2
correspondences, xiii
costs, 3, 12–13, 26, 51–52, 68
country, 3, 9, 64
court, 34, 61, 63
courtrooms, xiv
coverage, 13, 15, 17–20, 23, 29, 57, 63–64, 68, 71

covers, 9, 12
crashed, 8–9
created, xvii, 2–4, 33, 50, 59
customary, 8

D

damage, 40, 69
damaging, 14
deal, v, 8, 18, 20, 23, 35, 52–53
death and dismemberment, 37
debate, x–xvii, 2, 12, 14, 18, 59–61, 68–69, 71, 73
debt, 7
deceased, 56
decent, 8, 60
decided, 9
decision, 23, 50
declamation, 69
decriminalized, 7, 69
deductibles, 38–39
deduction, 63, 70
defending, x–xi
defenses, 25
deficits, 18
define, xvi, 36
degeneration, 37
degree, xv, 19, 25
delivered, 23, 53
delivery, xv
demanding, 57, 60
Democratic National Convention, xiv
Democratic Party, xi–xii, xvi, 7–8, 14, 19, 73–75
democratic system, 2, 71
Democrats, xi, 2, 13, 18–19
demotion, 34
dental, 9, 37–38, 40–41
Department of Administrative Services, 33–35, 41, 78
Department of Health Care Services (DHCS), 33
departments of health care, 3
depend, 15, 61–62
depends, xiv, 18
depressed, 45

describing, xii
description, 26–27, 72
deserved, 52
designations, 7
designed, 8, 59
design of errors, 27
despite, xiv
destruction, 7, 27
determination, v, 15, 25, 34
determined, 2, 25–26
developed, 8, 13, 24, 44
Dhore, xiii
Dhore, Hashi, xiii
differ, v, xiii, xv–xvii, 12–13, 18, 44–45, 60, 62, 71–72
different, xiii, xv–xvii, 12–13, 44, 62, 71–72
difficulties, 8, 23
diminishing, 28
diminution, 26, 38
diplomacies, 37
direction, xiii, 28, 37, 51, 71–75
directive, 59
directly, 20, 45
directors, 28
disability, 37, 40
disabled, 44, 47, 50
disadvantages, 26
disagreement, 7, 14, 26
discourse, xiii
discovered, 67
discretionary, 3
discussion, xiii
diseases, 12, 25
disinterested, 25, 44, 47
disparagement, 13
dispatch, 47
display, 34
disposition, 37–38, 40
dispossessed, 59
dissection, 15
dissimilar, 45
distasteful, 36

distinction, 25
distinguishing, 7
distributed, 24
distribution, 23, 26–27, 33, 50–51
division, 34–36, 41
doctors and hospitals, 8, 12
dollars, 4
donation, 28, 51
dosage, 45
dost deal, v
doubtingly, 46
Douthat, Ross, 18
down, xiv, 7, 9
during, xiii, 4, 7–8, 13, 45–46, 52, 68–70
duties, 44
duty commands, 35

E

easy, 13, 20, 23
easy-access, 20
edition, v–vi
education, xv, 12
effective, xv
effectively, x, xvi, 30, 68
effectiveness, 28
effects, 14
effort, xv, 4, 18, 24, 29–30, 35, 41, 58, 74
elected, 2, 73
electronic, 23
elements, 14
eligibility, 12–13
eligible, 9, 14, 20
embodies, 3
emolument, 35
employees, 33, 35
encouraged, 18, 47
encouragement, 27
engaged, xiii
engagement, 35–36, 52
engagements, 35
enhanced plan, 39

enhance e-health, 28
enrollment, 18
entire, xiv, 34–35, 41, 52
entitled, xii
equal, 36
equality, 2
equally, 18–19
equal opportunity, 36
equipment, 51, 53
especially, 14
established, 3, 27
European Union, 9, 73
evaluation, 28
examination, 24–25
examiner, 20, 78
exclusive, 56
exercises, 35
expanding, 13, 29, 68
expectation, 4
expected, 3, 20
expenditures, 23, 25, 38
expenses, 19, 51–52
expensive, 13, 18, 20, 23, 47, 57
experience, xiii, xvi, 73
experimental, 25
experts, 23, 41, 61
explained, xii
explosions, 51, 67
expression, 40
extensive, 27

G

Gaani, Sharmarke H., 33, 46–47
gas and mileage, 45
gathering, 35
gender or religion, 36
generate, 14, 23, 28, 35
gentlemen, 59
geology, xiv
God, v, xiii
governance, 24, 41, 78

government, 63
governor, 28
grandma, 62
Grand Old Party (GOP), 7, 19, 74
grants to programs, 59
great, 3, 7, 20, 23, 35, 52–53, 61
greatness, 12, 71
grieve, 56
gripped the nation, 59
grooming, 46
grow annually, 29
growing cost, 23
guaranteed, 58
guide, x
guiding, 3

H

Haberman, Maggie, 75
Hackman, Michelle, 70, 72
Haday, xvii
happening network, 39
harassment, 36
hard-wearing, 45, 75
hardworking, 4
harmful, 14, 69
Harvard Business School, 23
Hayes, Robert M., 57, 59
health care, xii, 2–4, 7–9, 12–15, 18–20, 23–26, 28, 30, 34, 36–38, 40, 44, 56–57, 68–75, 77–78
heart, 12, 14, 25, 62
heaviness, 46
heightening, 38
Heritage apartment, 60–61
Heritage community, 61
hidden, 19
higher costs, 3
higher-level, 8
highlighted, 47
highways, 67
history, xvii, 26, 67
home health care (HHC), 33–34, 36, 38, 41, 44, 47, 61, 63

home health-care communities, 50–51, 53
homeless citizens, 55–56
homelessness, 56–59
homoeopathic, 25
hooked, 39, 74
hospice care, 24, 62
house, 2–3, 7–9, 12–13, 67, 69, 73–75
household, 46, 60–61
House Minority, 8
House of Representatives, 2, 9, 13
House Republicans, 2
Housing and Urban Development (HUD), 58–59
How to Write Term Papers and Reports (Baugh), x, 77
Hughes, Shirley, 61
humanizing, 29
human resource, 3
human resources, 3, 32–36, 41
Human Resources Division (HRD), 33–36
humiliating, 72
hurting, 18–19
Hussien, Hawo, 60, 62
hypothetical, 27

I

identically, 36
identifiable, 29
identified, 74
ideology, 20
illustration, 25
imagine, x
immaculate, 62
immediate, 26
immigrants, 4, 50
impact, x, xiv, 7, 29
implemented, xii
important, 18, 57, 63
imports, 67
improved, 35, 38, 69
improvements, 35
inability, 60
inadequate, 59

incapacity, 40
incorporating, 24, 56, 72
incorporation, 33
increase, 2, 7, 20, 23, 26, 35
indicated, 8
indispensible, 35
individuals, 4, 23–24, 44, 59
industry, 3
infirmaries, 71
infirmary, 40
influence, 14, 52
influences, 25, 41
influential, 69
informality, xiv
information, x, xii, 47
inhabitants, 25, 72
initial, 57, 74
insisting, 7
inspections, 61
instead, x, xiv, 20
instigated, 74
institute, 24, 58
institutional, 3
institutions, 12, 47
instruction, 23, 34, 71
insurance, 4, 8, 13–15, 22, 63, 66, 68, 70
intellectual, 8
intelligent, 56
intensification, 36, 39, 52
intensifications, 52
intensify, 23, 39
intensifying, 23
interested, 9, 18
Internal Revenue Service (IRS), 50
interpersonal, 33
interpretations, 36
introductions, 45
investigate, 63
investigation, 29, 41, 47, 74
investigator, 18
investments, 67

involving, 27
Iraq, 4, 56, 59, 75

K

Kaar, Cali, xvii
Kaiser Family Foundation, 73
keen, 45
Keisha, xiv
Kennedy, John F., 75
Kenya, 62
kept, 7
key, 50
killing, 67
kindhearted, 67
Kingdom, 9
kinship, 46
knocking, 44
knowledge, x, 73
Korean War, 56
Krow, Shailynn, 44
Kulan, Basro, 60, 62–63

L

Lucas, Stephen, xiii

M

maintain, 3, 60, 73
maintenance, 51
majorities, 2
major social, 57
makers, 50
Malia, 62
management, 23, 28, 35
manager, 33–34, 61
mannerisms, xv
manners, x, 26
margin, 19
marginally, 25
Maricopa, 25
marketplace, 14
married couple, 29

Mary Catholic Church, 62
massive, 24
material, 53
materialization, 56
matter, 8
matters, 26
maximum, xiv, 40
maximum impact, xiv
mayors, 59
McCarthy, Carolyn, xiv
McKinney, 58
McKinney-Vento Homeless Assistance Act, 58
measurements, 23, 56
Medicade and Medicare, 7, 9
Medicaid, 8–9, 13–14, 19–20, 56–57, 64, 68, 72, 78
Medi-Cal, 71
medical treatment, 4
Medicare, 7–9, 12–13, 19, 24–25, 68, 71
medications, 45
members, 4, 67, 74
memberships, 8
memo, 14
memorize, x
mental, 25, 63
merely, x
messenger, v
method, xv, 27
middle-income families, 13–14, 68
million, 13, 15, 18, 59–60, 68
minimum, 35, 40
minority, 8
miscalculations, 28
miserly, v
Mitch M., 67
model, 28, 30
modern, 41
modification, 23
Mohamed, Ismail, xiii
momentousness, 67
moral cost, xvii, 56
moralities, 68

motionlessly, 4
movement, 19
MSNBC, 8
municipal, xi
municipality, 73
Muslim-majority, 74

N

narrate, 51
national, xiv, 57, 59, 77
national government, 2, 4
National Visitors Center, 57
nation's 45 million, 13
necessary, x, xv, 3–4, 20, 53
necessity, 12
negatively, xv
negative note, 3
newfangled, 38
new hire, 34–35, 44
New York Times, 18, 75, 78
non-preferred, 40
non-profit, 50
normal, 25, 61
Northern Rock, 24
NPR analysis, 73
number of citizens, 19
numerous, 7, 23, 29, 36
nurses, 33, 39, 44–47

O

Obama, Barack, 2, 8, 12, 18, 59, 62, 71, 73
Obama, Michele, 62
Obama administration, 4, 6–7, 9, 19, 71, 74–75
Obama Care, x–xii, xvi–xvii, 4, 7–9, 14–15, 18–20, 24, 50, 55–57, 63–64, 68–71, 73–75, 77
ObamaCare, 77
Office of Collective Bargaining (OCB), 33
Ohio, xiii, 33–36, 38, 41, 44–46, 50–51, 60–61
operating, 34
operational, 40
opinions, 12, 18

opportunity, 36
oppose, 4
opposing, 2, 13
oppositional, 36
oppositions, xi
organizations, 2–3, 9, 20, 24, 29, 36, 50–51, 78
organizing, xiii
originally, 7, 56
originate, 33, 75

P

Pelosi, Nancy, 8
Peterson, Kristina, 70, 72
Prices, Rita, 47
Public Sector-Third Sector, 24

R

Rankin, Kristen, 33–35
Reagan, Ronald W., 58
reason, xii
re-authorization, 14
recommendation, 25, 47, 72
recommended, 35
recovered, 25–26, 45
referendum, 58
reformed, 2, 7
regardless, 29
registered, 9, 44, 50
regularity, 26
rehabilitation, 45
reimbursements, 38
rejection, xvi, 38
repayments, 25–26, 37
repeal and replace, xii
reports, x, 77
representatives, 2, 7, 9, 13, 75
Republican Party, xi–xii, xvii, 2–4, 7, 9, 18, 68–69, 72, 75
Republicans, 2, 4, 7–9, 13–15, 18, 20, 63, 67, 71, 73
required, 46–47, 60, 68, 70
requires, xiv, 12, 71
research, x, 18, 51

reservation, 56
resolution, xii
resources, 32, 34–36, 41
respectable, 38, 47
respective, 25, 45, 70
restructuring, 13
reviewing, 33
RN, 27
roadmap in Arizona, 22

S

Safari Coffee, xiii
safety and training, 34
satisfactory, 53
Section 8 Housing, 58
separately, 33
sequestered, 8, 36, 73
sexual harassment, 36
shelter, 8, 19, 56–60, 71
short-time disability, 37
sicknesses, 25
slang, jargon, xiv
Snyder, Mitch, 57
Somalia, xiii, xvi–xvii, 56, 61–63, 73, 75
speaker of debate, xi
spearhead, 8
specimen, 36
Srivastava, Kalpana, 3, 78
statement, x, xii, 12, 36
strengthened, 19
strenuously, 36
stretched, 19
struggled, 8
struggling to steer, 68
stylishness, 45
subject, x
subsidies, 13–14, 60, 68
substandard, 71
Sumaca, xvii
summarized, 29
superficially, 24

supplementary, 37, 46, 72
Supreme Court of American, xi
sustenance, vi, xvi
systematically, xiii, 75

T

tailoring, xiv
tasteless, 45–46
Taylor, James Stacey, 2, 29
Taylor, Jessica, 73
Tea party movement, 19
techniques, 28, 34–35, 71
tensions, 20
terminated, 37
therapeutic, 45
threatened, 7, 58, 61
Thrush, Glenn, 75
Tim Horton's, xvii
tolerate, 36
trademark, 38
training health care workers, 13
transformations, 35, 37, 47
transforming, 38, 77
transition, 28
translation, v–vi
transporter, 38
travel and conference, 51
traveling, 44, 47
Travers, Karen, 62
treasuries, 36
treatments, 4, 9, 12, 20, 37, 44–45
trillion, 7
trooped, 26
"Trouble with Champions," 24, 78
Trump, Donald, xii, 18, 67–68, 70, 73–75
Tyler, Andrew, 60
typically, 36, 44

W

Wagner, 68
Wall Street Journal, 70, 72
Wall Street law, 59
warrants, 35
Washington Post, 9, 69–70, 73, 78
Welker, Kristen, 8
wert, v
Whitecanos and White, x, xii, 36
White House, 8, 12, 67, 73–75

www.ingramcontent.com/pod-product-compliance
Lightning Source LLC
Chambersburg PA
CBHW030845180526
45163CB00004B/1450